STEP-BY-

MASSAGE

FOR PAIN RELIEF

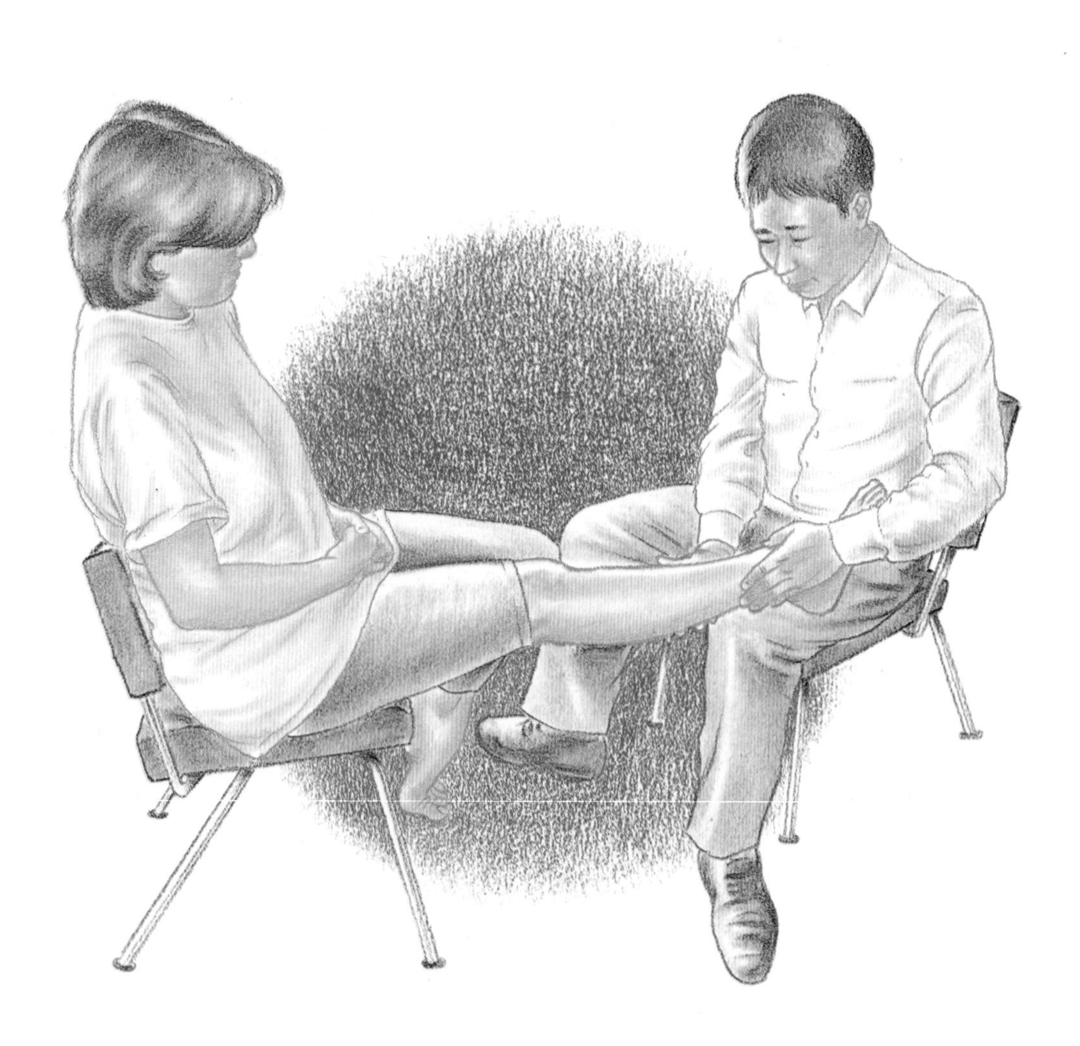

STEP-BY-STEP

MASSAGE

FOR PAIN RELIEF

by
Peijian Shen

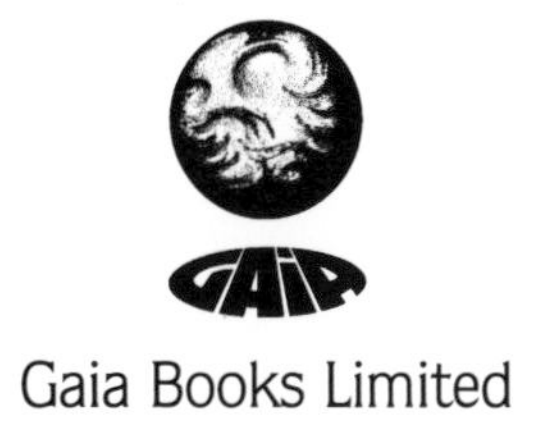

Gaia Books Limited

A GAIA ORIGINAL

Books from Gaia celebrate the vision of Gaia, the self-sustaining living Earth, and seek to help its readers live in greater personal and planetary harmony.

Editor	Fiona Trent
Designer	Kitty Parker-Jervis
Illustrators	Aziz Khan, Tim Monk, Helen Ward
Managing Editor	Pip Morgan
Production	Susan Walby
Direction	Joss Pearson, Patrick Nugent

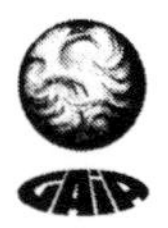

This edition published in 2000
First published in the United Kingdom in 1996 by
Gaia Books Ltd, 66 Charlotte St, London W1P 1LR
and 20 High St, Stroud, Glos GL5 1AS

ISBN 1 85675 131 7

A catalogue record of this book is available from the British Library.

Printed and bound by MRM Graphics in Singapore

10 9 8 7 6 5 4 3 2 1

This book is not intended to replace medical care under the direct supervision of a qualified doctor. Before embarking on any changes in your health regime, consult your doctor.

Gaia Books would like to thank: Helena Petre, Eleanor Lines, and Charlie Ryrie for editorial assistance; Mary Warren for compiling the index; Helena Petre, Jenny Banfield, Helen Conway-Jones, Owen Elias, Sam Bloomfield, Gilda, and Katherine Pate for acting as models.

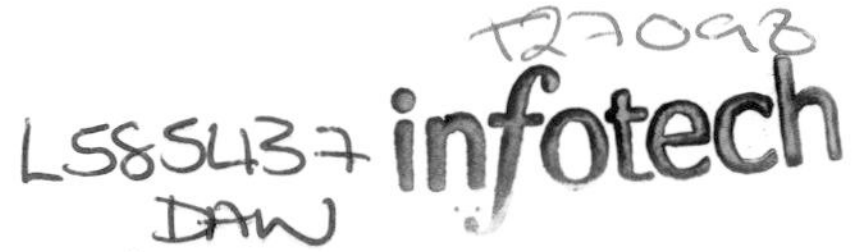

CONTENTS

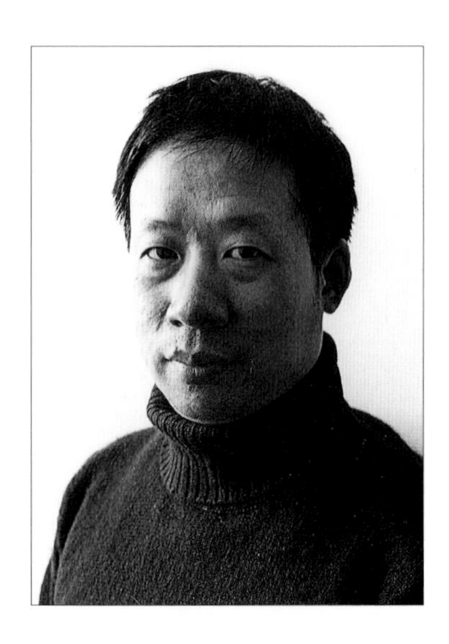

A note from the author

As a child I frequently received Chinese massage and acupuncture due to my own disability, caused by polio. I understood how disease and pain caused people to suffer, and how much these therapies mean to such people. I learned to practise Chinese massage therapy under a relative's tuition, and continued my studies at medical school, where I worked with the masters of Chinese massage. The method described in this book is based on my own experience, and that of traditional Chinese massage practitioners.

Pain-relief massage is a technique taken from Chinese massage. I have written this book for anyone interested in the therapy, whatever your previous experience and knowledge. Massage for pain relief aims to open stagnated Channels and to smooth energy circulation in the body, by working on the Channels, key acupoints, and pain-relief points. It is an easy and effective method of relieving painful disorders of various kinds, and doesn't have any side effects. It can also play an important role in the rehabilitation process after injury or surgery. Pain-relief massage is effective in overcoming fatigue, helping people to relax, and in promoting individual health and wellbeing. Generally, it has a favourable effect on the circulatory, nervous, respiratory, digestive, urogenital, and immune systems, as well as on the endocrine and motor functions. You can practise this method on its own or with other therapies.

How to use this book

The book is made up of an Introduction, four chapters, and an Appendix. The Introduction explains the basic theory of Chinese medicine. Chapter One presents a simple, easy-to-use self-care massage programme, which you should practise daily to maintain and improve your own health and wellbeing. Chapter Two describes the various massage techniques, and some basic rules of practice. Chapter Three concentrates on the method of opening the Channels in the various regions of the body, an approach that is still relatively unknown to those practising alternative medicine in the West. Chapter Four shows you how to apply the massage techniques you have learned to bring about pain relief for a wide range of conditions. You can also use these treatments as reference information for treating pain caused by other similar diseases or conditions. The Appendix includes detailed information about the course of each Channel, and the symptoms of disease typical to each Channel. Detailed information on the location and function of all the acupoints referred to in this book is also given in the Appendix.

If you are new to Chinese medicine, and have any initial difficulty with this book, put your questions aside, and continue to read and practise. With experience and a growing understanding, you will soon find that the "difficulty" is not as great as it used to be. This highly illustrated, step-by-step book makes pain-relief massage easy to learn. Remember that practice is the best teacher you can have – with time it will bring you success.

I would like to thank the many people who have helped in the writing of this book. I wish to thank Miss Jenny Crichton, Miss Jen Beales, Ms C. Kerr-Dineen, and Mr Stephen Garton for their help with the revised text. In addition, my thanks are naturally due to my friend Shigeo Ushimaru, and to my sister Shen Yanzhi. The manuscript could not have been completed without their assistance in drawing reference illustrations.

Peijian Shen ~ 1995

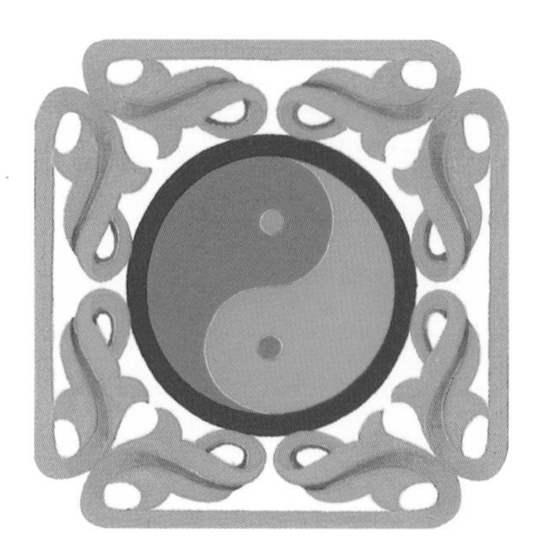

INTRODUCTION

Chinese massage, like acupuncture and herbal medicine, has been effectively used to cure disease in China for some 2000 years. Massage for pain relief is a form of Chinese massage. It is a natural and physical therapy that works on Channels, acupoints, pain-relief points, and affected parts of the body with various manipulations to relieve symptoms of pain and cure disease. It follows the fundamental rule of Chinese medicine, namely, that "to cure disease, you must cure its root". To understand how pain-relief massage works, we first need an understanding of the some of the basic concepts of Chinese medicine.

Yin and Yang

Traditional Chinese medicine offers us a unique and exclusive answer to the age-old questions "What is life?" and "How is life created?" Its simple suggestion is that life is the connection of Yin and Yang. Yin and Yang create life by touching each other: they are the basis of all life.

Yin and Yang are the opposite aspects of matter and phenomena in nature, but they are complementary and interdependent. The Yin-Yang principle is the basis of the theory and practice of traditional Chinese medicine. Everything in the universe has Yin and Yang characteristics. For example, all aspects of the human body can be divided into Yin and Yang, and when in full health the two forces are in perfect balance.

Qi and blood

Two essential substances, namely Qi and blood, are needed to support life. Qi, in a narrow sense, refers to vital energy – the primary motive force of all activities of life. Qi has two fundamental functions – to nourish the body, and to protect it from external damage. It is usually accompanied by blood. Qi and blood support and complement each other: blood needs Qi to keep it moving, and Qi needs blood to generate it. According to Chinese medicine, "Qi is the leader of Blood; Blood is the mother of Qi". Qi and blood circulate together through the Channels as "Qi-blood flow". In normal, healthy conditions, Qi-blood should flow smoothly. However, if the flow is disturbed, Qi and blood stagnate in the Channels, and block them, which sometimes causes pain.

What causes Qi-blood stagnation?

Traditional Chinese medicine tells us that there are Six Evils, or external pathogenic factors, that can upset Qi-blood flow. They are Wind, Cold, Summer-heat, Damp, Dryness, and Fire. Normally, our bodies can adapt to small changes in these factors, but if one or more are in excess, or in short supply, Qi disturbance and stagnation may occur.

Stagnation can also result from internal pathogenic factors, such as an irregular lifestyle, exhaustion, and an excess of the Seven Extreme Emotions. These are over-excitement, anxiety, anger, worry, grief, fear, and shock. If in excess, any one of these emotions can disturb the function of the Viscera, and upset the balance of Yin and Yang, and Qi-blood flow.

The Viscera

In traditional Chinese medicine the term Viscera refers to three groups of organs (see right): the Zang organs, which are Yin; the Fu organs, which are Yang; and the Extraordinary organs. The Viscera are linked by the Channel system (see pp. 10-11).

The Viscera have a wider meaning in Chinese medicine than organs do in Western thinking. For example, in Chinese medicine, the kidney is responsible not only for water metabolism, but also for providing a link between sources of energy and growth, the bones and brain. For this reason, the Chinese concept of an organ will be presented throughout this book with an initial capital letter – Kidney – to differentiate it from the strict anatomical meaning used in the West.

The Viscera groups

The three organ groups which make up the Viscera are shown below.

☆ The Pericardium is sometimes included as a Zang organ. As an organ it merely assists the Heart, but it has its own Channel.

★ The Triple Warmer is not a true organ, it is the passageway for Qi and fluids through the abdomen. It has three segments: the Upper, Middle, and Lower Warmer.

Fu organs
Small Intestine
Gall Bladder
Stomach
Large Intestine
Urinary Bladder
★Triple Warmer

Zang organs
Heart
Liver
Spleen
Lungs
Kidney
☆ Pericardium

Extraordinary organs
Brain
Bone marrow
Bone
Blood vessels
Uterus
Gall Bladder

The Channel system

A system of Channels, through which Qi and blood flow, was precisely described in the first Chinese medical book *Nei Jing* (Canon of Medicine) more than 2000 years ago. The system consists of 12 Regular Channels, 8 Extra Channels, and some collaterals. In this book we discuss the Channels most commonly used in treatment. These are the Regular Channels and two of the Extra Channels – Du and Ren.

The Regular Channels are distributed symmetrically on both sides of the body. They connect to each other to form a continuous circuit. Each Regular Channel also connects with one of the internal Viscera (see p. 9). The Channel system serves to integrate the Viscera, limbs, and all other parts of the body including the bones, muscles, tendons, and skin into one whole. The Channels also help to balance the Yin and Yang of the Viscera.

If any of the Six Evils or the Seven Extreme Emotions invade the body (see p. 9), or if there is a problem with any of the Viscera, the Channels will be disturbed and Qi-blood flow disrupted. This is referred to as Channel blockage, or Qi-blood stagnation. The Channels and Viscera may lose the balance of Yin and Yang. Channel disturbance may be manifested in certain parts of the body as external signs and symptoms of disease such as pain.

Yin Channels of the Hand	**Yang Channels of the Hand**
Lung Channel of Hand ~ *Taiyin*	Large Intestine Channel of Hand ~ *Yangming*
Pericardium Channel of Hand ~ *Jueyin*	Triple Warmer Channel of Hand ~ *Shoyang*
Heart Channel of Hand ~ *Shaoyin*	Small Intestine Channel of Hand ~ *Taiyang*
Yang Channels of the Foot	**Yin Channels of the Foot**
Stomach Channel of Foot ~ *Yangming*	Spleen Channel of Foot ~ *Taiyin*
Gall Bladder Channel of Foot ~ *Shoyang*	Liver Channel of Foot ~ *Jueyin*
Urinary Bladder Channel of Foot ~ *Taiyang*	Kidney Channel of Foot ~ *Shaoyin*

Names of the Regular Channels

Each of the 12 Regular Channels connects with one of the internal organs, follows a course along either the arm or the leg, and is associated with either Yin or Yang. The full Chinese name for each Channel is made up of these three components (see chart, left). However, for simplicity, in the rest of this book we will refer to the Channels by their organ name only.

Qi-blood flow

This illustration represents the movement of Qi and blood through the Channels. Qi and blood start their circuit in the Lung Channel, and flow through the other Channels one by one in a fixed Yin-Yang order. Qi and blood finally return to the Lung Channel, where the cycle begins again. The exact course of each individual Channel is given in the Appendix (see pp. 122-27).

The Yin Channels converge in the abdomen; all the Yang Channels meet in the head region. Each Channel meets its paired Channel at either the hand or the foot.

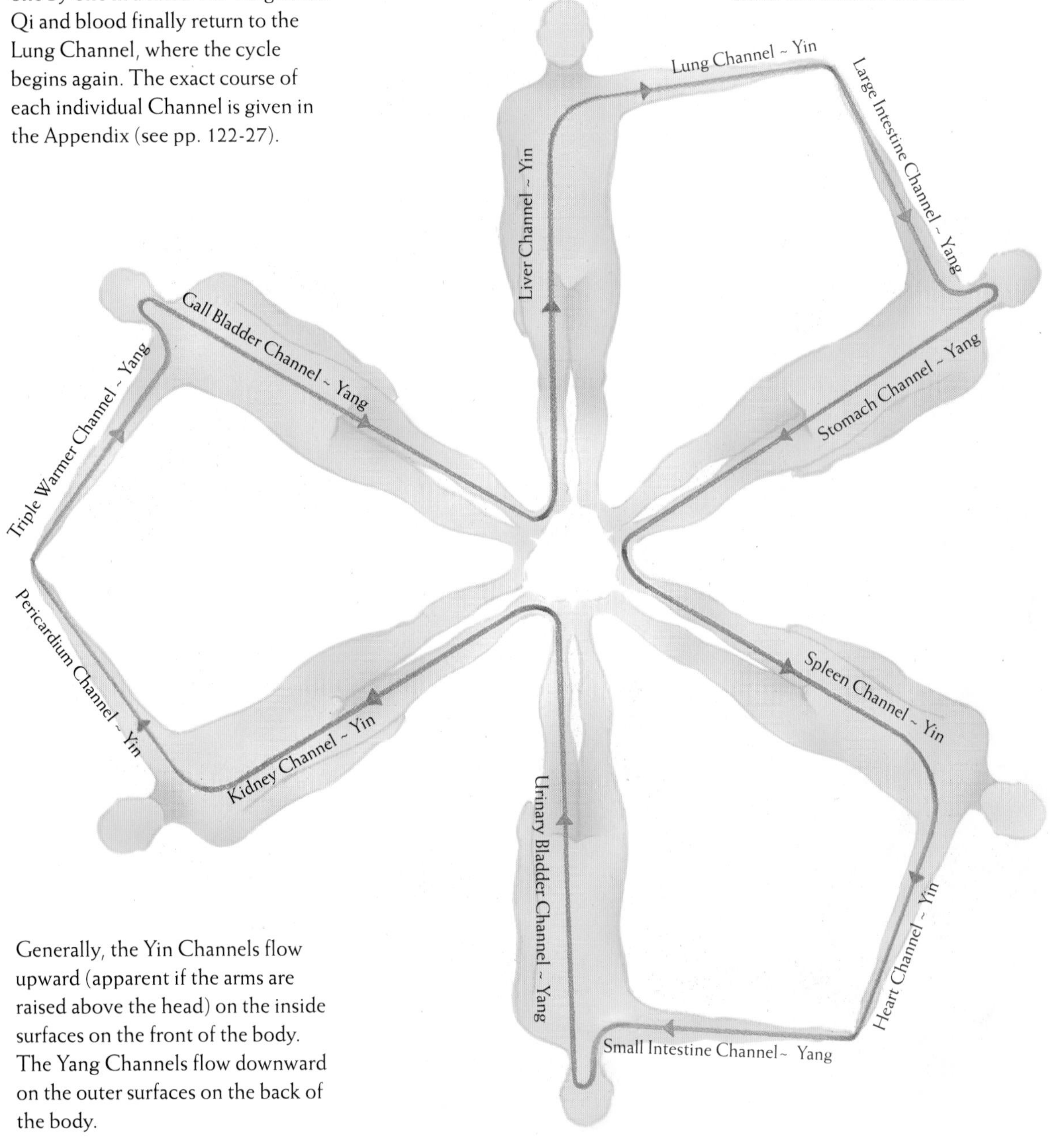

Generally, the Yin Channels flow upward (apparent if the arms are raised above the head) on the inside surfaces on the front of the body. The Yang Channels flow downward on the outer surfaces on the back of the body.

Pain-relief massage

The exact site of a symptom reflects which Channel is disturbed, and which organ is affected by disease. For example, pain in the rib area often signifies disease of the Liver or Gall Bladder, and pain in the collarbone area is likely to reflect a Lung problem. Refer to the Appendix (see pp. 122-27) for the most common symptoms of disturbance for each Channel.

The association between symptoms and Channel disturbance forms the basis for pain-relief massage treatment. By massaging the relevant Channels, acupoints, and carefully chosen pain-relief points, pain is relieved. Pain-relief massage achieves this by removing Qi-blood stagnation, opening the Channels, and restoring the balance of Yin and Yang. Pain-relief massage can ease pain not only on the surface of the body, but also in the internal organs, because the Channel network links the exterior of the body to the interior. Massage of points on the surface of the body affects the internal organs too.

Interior	**Exterior**
Lung Channel	Large Intestine Channel
Spleen Channel	Stomach Channel
Heart Channel	Small Intestine Channel
Kidney Channel	Urinary Bladder Channel
Pericardium Channel	Triple Warmer Channel
Liver Channel	Gall Bladder Channel
Yin	**Yang**

Channel pairs

The 12 Regular Channels separate into six pairs. One of each pair is Yang, the other Yin, and together they form an exterior-interior relationship. Each Channel joins its corresponding partner at the end of a limb (see p. 11) and each pair lie symmetrically, one on either side of the limb. The organs associated with these Channels also have an exterior-interior relationship.

Acupoints

The word "acupoint" in Chinese means a small hole for Qi. Hundreds of acupoints lie along the course of the Channels, and they help to transmit Qi and blood through the Channels. They are closely related to the Viscera, and to all parts of the body, and they reflect physiological and pathological changes in the body. Acupoints are massaged to regulate Qi-blood flow and the functioning of the Viscera.

There are two types of acupoint: the normal acupoints, which lie on the Regular Channels, and on the Du and Ren Channels, and the extraordinary acupoints, which are not located on a Channel. In addition, there are some points, known as pain-relief points, which can be classified either as normal acupoints or as extraordinary acupoints. Pain-relief points, as their name suggests, have the specific function of relieving pain in certain parts of the body. The central point of an area of pain, known as the pain-pressure point, is also a type of pain-relief point.

In this book, we use a Chinese name and a code name for each acupoint. The Chinese name often explains the acupoint's function. For example, *Feishu* literally means "point related to the Lung". However, in the West, the code names are preferred. The code is composed of an abbreviation of the Channel and a number relating to the position of the acupoint along its Channel. For example, UB13 (the code for *Feishu*) indicates the 13th point along the Urinary Bladder Channel. The abbreviations of the Channels are given in the Appendix (see p. 128), as are details of the location and application of all the acupoints mentioned in this book (see pp. 128-39).

General caution

Massage is a safe and reliable method for pain relief. However, it would be wrong to perceive this therapy as an all-purpose cure, since it is not universally applicable. For example, do not massage pregnant women, or anyone who is either very infirm or extremely nervous. Avoid massaging a woman's lower back and hips during menstruation, and do not apply massage immediately after someone has been treated with acupuncture or a hot compress.

Do not apply massage in any of the following situations:

- fractures or dislocations
- infectious diseases
- during the critical or acute stage of a disease – for example, when there is a high fever
- in cases of excessively high blood pressure or a cardiac infection
- in cases of skin problems such as serious dermatitis and abscesses
- malignant tumours and scrofula
- in cases of internal haemorrhage

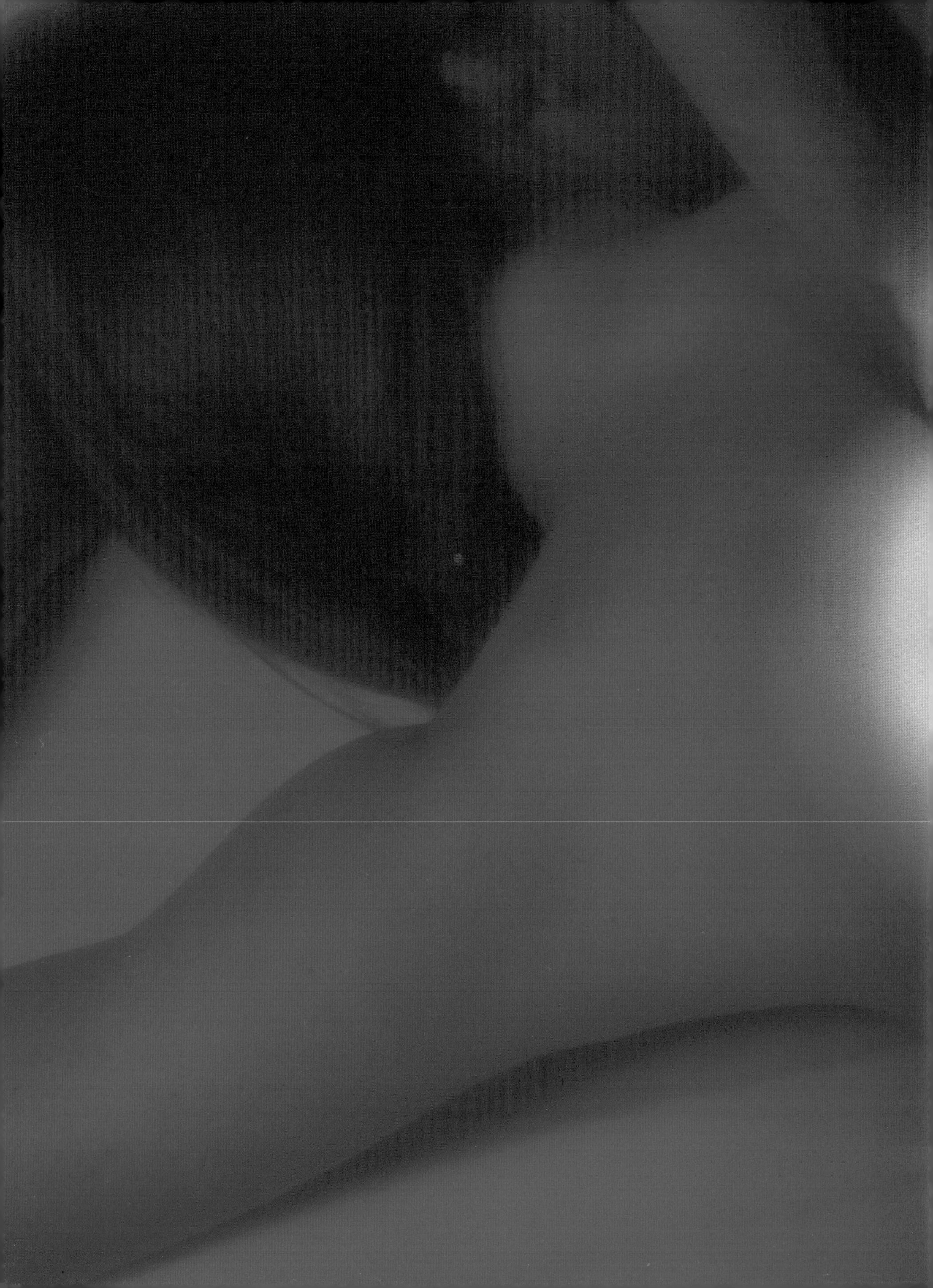

part one

THE FOUNDATIONS

CHAPTER ONE

SELF-CARE MASSAGE

A WELL-KNOWN CHINESE PROVERB STATES THAT "A MEDIOCRE DOCTOR CURES DISEASE WHEREAS A GOOD DOCTOR PREVENTS IT." THIS VIEW IS FUNDAMENTAL TO CHINESE MEDICINE WHERE PREVENTION RATHER THAN CURE IS THE PRIME CONSIDERATION.

MASSAGE IS ONE WAY TO PREVENT ILL HEALTH AND DISEASE. MASSAGE IS USUALLY GIVEN BY ONE PERSON TO ANOTHER, BUT YOU CAN ALSO PRACTISE IT ON YOURSELF. SELF-CARE MASSAGE IS A SIMPLE AND EFFECTIVE TECHNIQUE THAT ALMOST EVERYONE CAN USE (SEE P.13 FOR EXCEPTIONS).

THIS SELF-CARE MASSAGE ROUTINE IS PRESENTED AS A SERIES OF DIAGRAMS AND INSTRUCTIONS. YOU CAN EITHER PERFORM THE FULL SEQUENCE TO IMPROVE YOUR OVERALL HEALTH AND WELL-BEING, OR CONCENTRATE ON SPECIFIC EXERCISES TO HELP ALLEVIATE A PARTICULAR PROBLEM. IF YOU ARE IN PAIN, YOU SHOULD IDEALLY SEEK PAIN-RELIEF MASSAGE FIRST (SEE PP. 66-121), AND FOLLOW THIS WITH SELF-CARE MASSAGE TO CONTINUE THE IMPROVEMENT. HOWEVER, SELF-CARE MASSAGE WILL ALSO HELP IF PERFORMED ON ITS OWN. REFER TO CHAPTER TWO (SEE PP. 28-45) FOR FURTHER INFORMATION ON THE MASSAGE STROKES REFERRED TO IN THIS CHAPTER.

AIM TO GIVE YOURSELF ABOUT A FIFTEEN-MINUTE SELF-CARE MASSAGE EVERY DAY TO PROMOTE GOOD GENERAL PHYSICAL AND EMOTIONAL HEALTH.

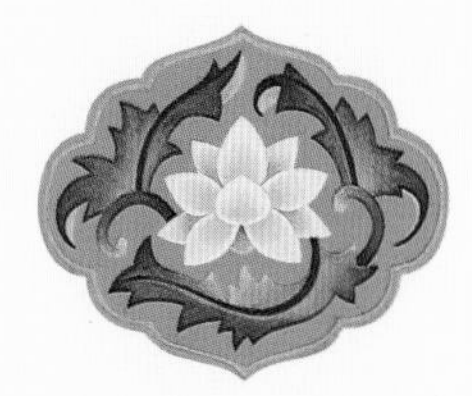

SELF-CARE MASSAGE OF THE HEAD AND FACE

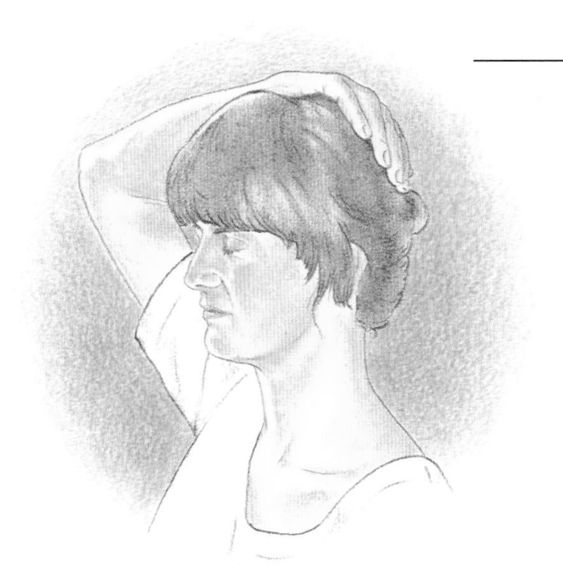

Kneading the head

Place the heel of your right hand on the top of your head, midway between your ears. This covers the acupoint known as Du20 (*Baihui*). Apply moderate pressure and knead the area slowly with 10 circular clockwise strokes, and then 10 anti-clockwise strokes.

In Chinese medicine the brain is called the "Reservoir of Marrow". Du20 (see p. 128) is the key acupoint that controls the flow of Qi passing through the reservoir. This massage therefore has a beneficial effect on the brain. It also enhances the memory, and prevents high blood pressure.

Kneading the temples

Put your thumbs either side of your face on the temples, one thumb-width away from the outside edge of the eye and level with the top of the ear. This is the position of the extra acupoints known as *Taiyang*. Knead both points slowly in a clockwise direction and with moderate pressure. Repeat 30 times.

Taiyang (see p. 129) is very effective in treating a variety of disorders in the head region. This massage helps to prevent headaches, insomnia, and eye problems such as short-sightedness. It also relaxes the brain.

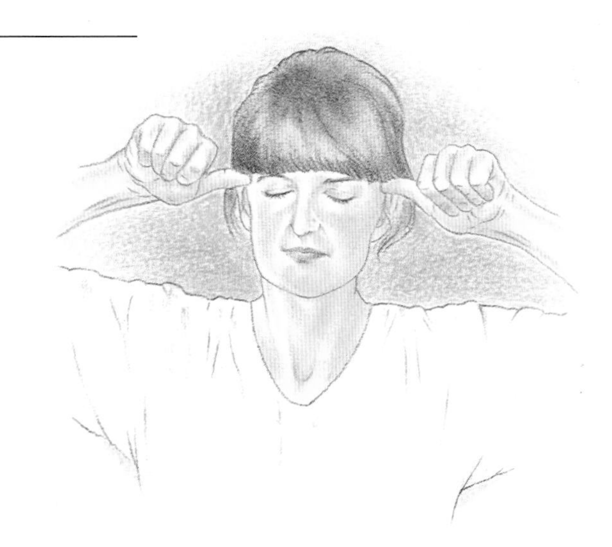

Combing the head

Let your fingers curl naturally. Then, using your fingertips, apply moderate pressure and comb your head from the forehead hair line to the back of the neck. Repeat 20 times.

All the Yang Channels meet in the head, which in Chinese medicine is called the "Converging Place of all Yang". This massage relaxes the brain, improves the memory, and prevents neurosis.

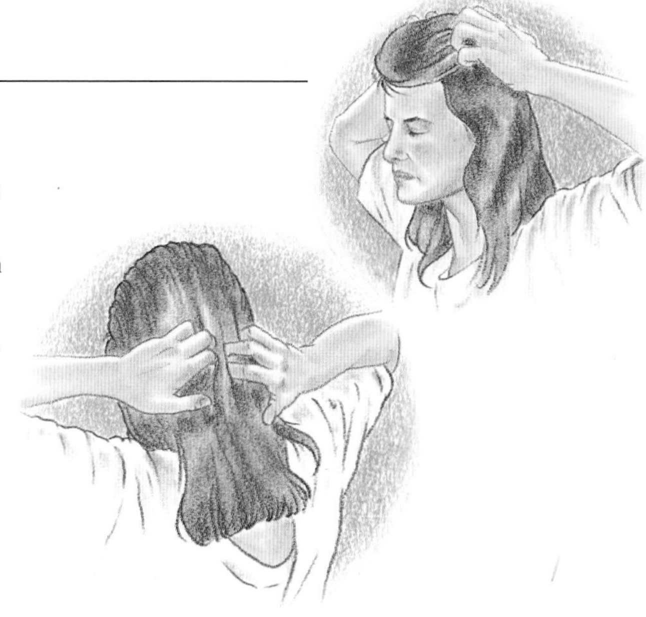

Pushing the eyebrows

Place the tips of your middle fingers on the inner ends of your eyebrows. Then, with gentle pressure, push along your eyebrows to their outer ends. Repeat 10 times.

This simple massage stimulates three acupoints along the eyebrow. It relaxes the eyes, and prevents eye diseases and headaches.

Rotating the eyes

Close your eyes and slowly rotate your eyeballs clockwise three times and then anticlockwise three times. Repeat three times and then open your eyes and look ahead to finish the sequence. Repeat the whole sequence three times.

In Chinese medicine the eyes are called the "Doors of Life". This exercise relaxes the eyes and keeps them in good condition.

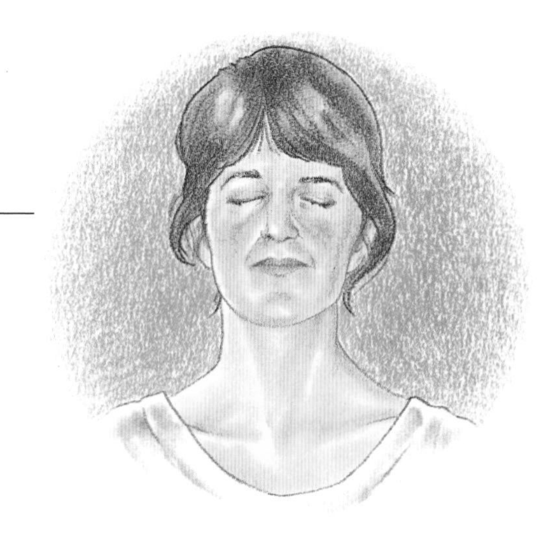

Wiping the face

Rub your hands together until they are warm. Then place your palms either side of your nose and slide them across your cheeks toward the ears with a smooth, wiping action. Massage your face in this way 10 times.

This gentle massage increases the circulation of blood to the face. It also improves the elasticity of the skin and helps to prevent wrinkles.

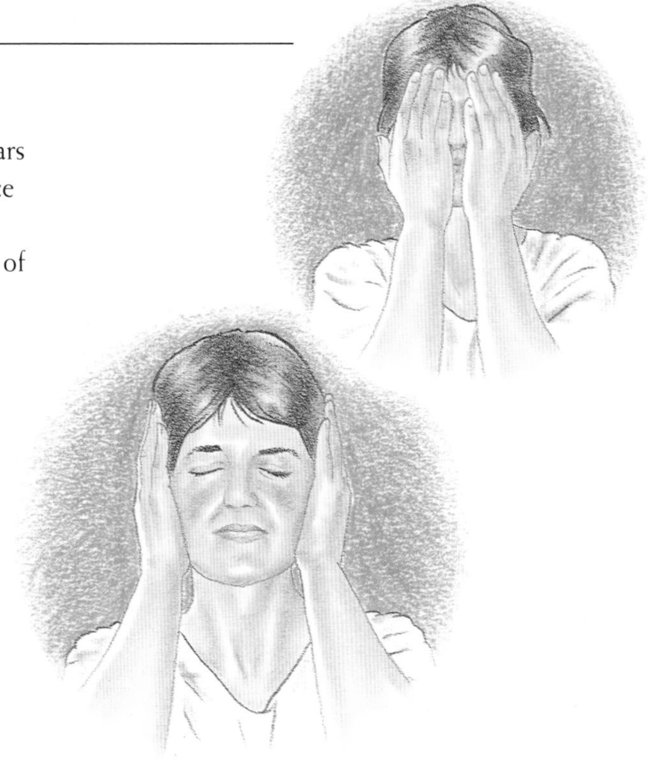

CAUTION
DO NOT PERFORM THIS MASSAGE IF YOU SUFFER FROM ACNE OR PIMPLES.

Pushing the nose

Place your index fingers on either side of the bridge of your nose. Push down the sides of your nose toward the nostrils. Apply moderate pressure and speed, and repeat the stroke 20 times.

This massage, which in Chinese is called "Pushing the Life Longer", stimulates several acupoints including LI20 (*Yingxiang*) (see p. 120). Use this massage to prevent respiratory disorders.

Pinching the ears

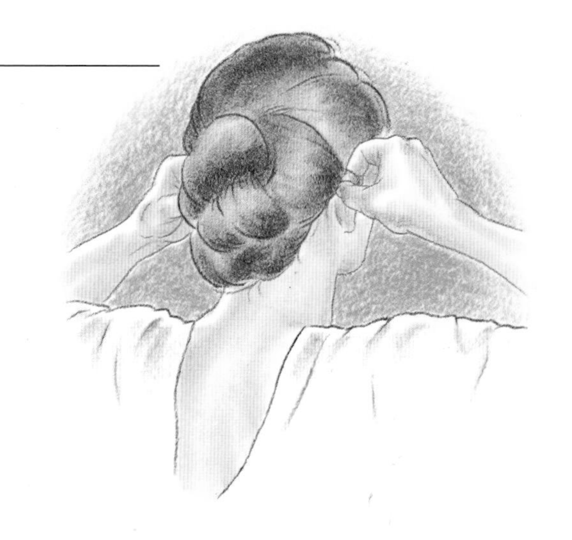

Remove any earrings before you start this massage. With your thumbs and index fingers, pinch your ears with moderate pressure. Start at the top of your ear and work down to the lobes. Repeat 10 times.

The ears are home to numerous acupoints, which relate to all the other organs and parts of the body. This massage, by stimulating your whole ear, benefits your overall health. More specifically, it also prevents high blood pressure.

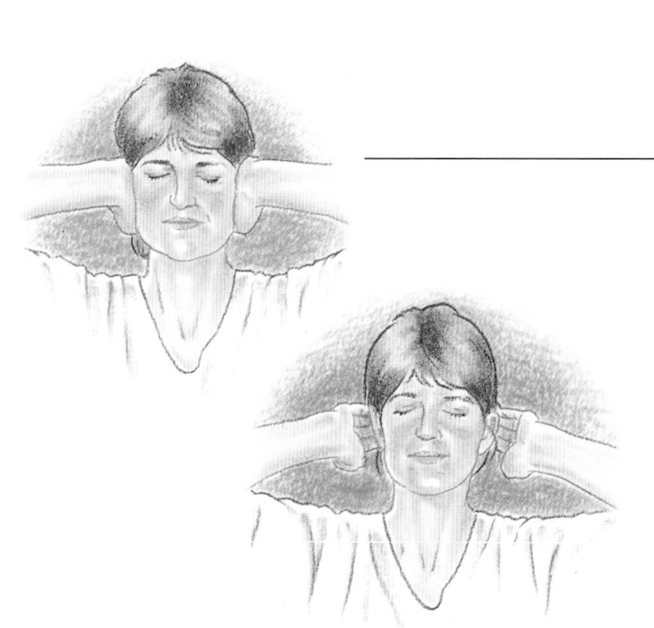

Pressing the ears

Place your palms over your ears with your fingers pointing toward the back of your head. Press your palms down tightly and then remove them quickly. When you remove your palms, you may hear a sound like a drumbeat. Repeat 10 times.

This exercise improves your hearing and prevents various ear diseases, particularly tinnitus.

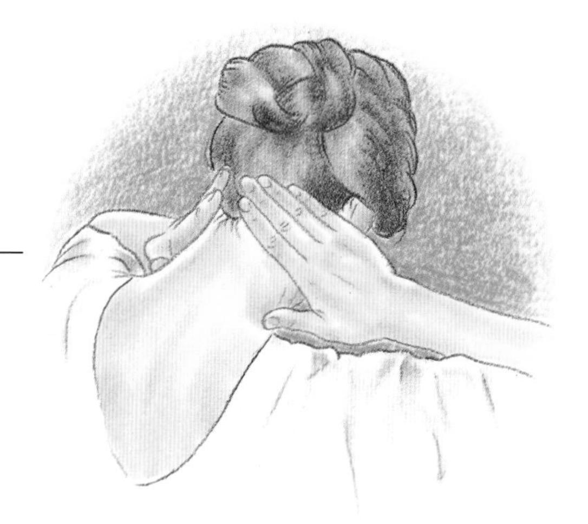

Rubbing the neck

Place your palms behind your ears on the back of your neck. This covers both GB20 (*Fengchi*) acupoints, either side of the head (see p. 129). With your palms, rub back and forth over the acupoints 30 times. The rubbing action may make your neck feel warm.

This massage helps to prevent the onset of the common cold.

SELF-CARE MASSAGE OF THE ABDOMEN AND BACK

Kneading the breastbone

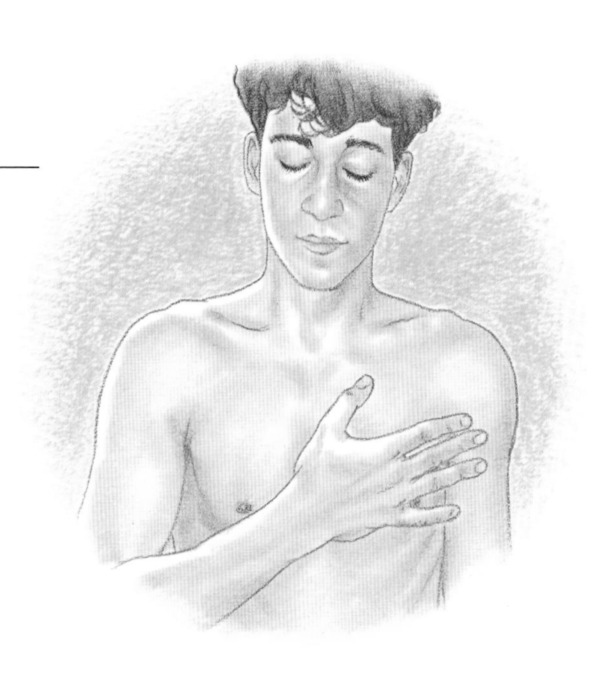

Place the heel of your right hand on your breastbone, midway between the nipples. This is the position of the acupoint Ren17 (*Tanzhong*). Apply moderate pressure and knead the area with 40 alternating clockwise and anticlockwise circles.

Ren17 (see p. 131) is related to the Pericardium. It is also known as the "Reservoir of Qi" because Qi collects there. This massage benefits the Heart, and other organs such as the Liver and Spleen.

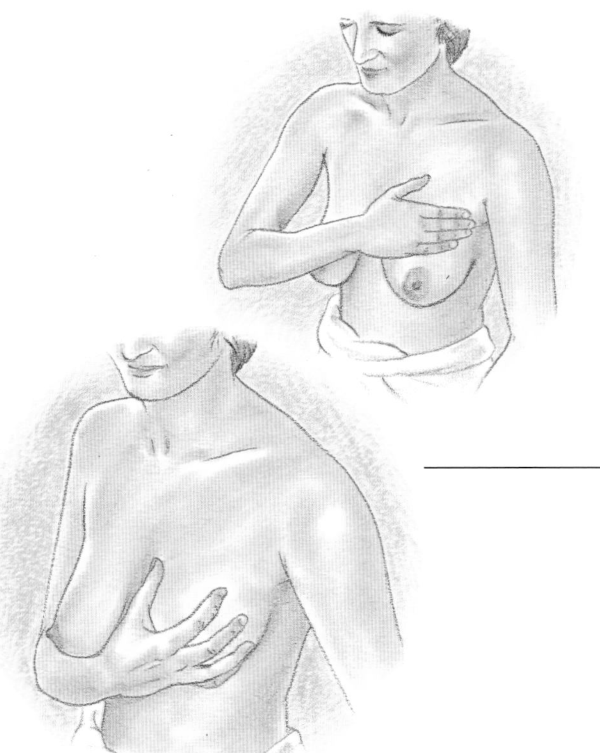

CAUTION
DO NOT PRACTISE MASSAGE IN THE ABDOMINAL REGION IF YOU ARE PREGNANT.

Kneading the breasts

With the palm of your right hand, rub around your left breast 20 times. Change hands and rub around your right breast 20 times. Then cup your left breast in your right hand, squeeze gently, and quickly release 20 times. Repeat the squeezing sequence on your right breast 20 times.

Massaging the breasts in this way helps to keep them in good physical condition.

Circling around the navel

Before you start, rub your palms together in a relaxed and purposeful way to warm them. Then place your right palm on your abdomen and rub a clockwise circle around the navel. Repeat 20 times, applying a little more pressure each time.

This massage stimulates many of the acupoints and Channels in the abdominal area and improves Qi-blood flow. Apply it to improve your digestion.

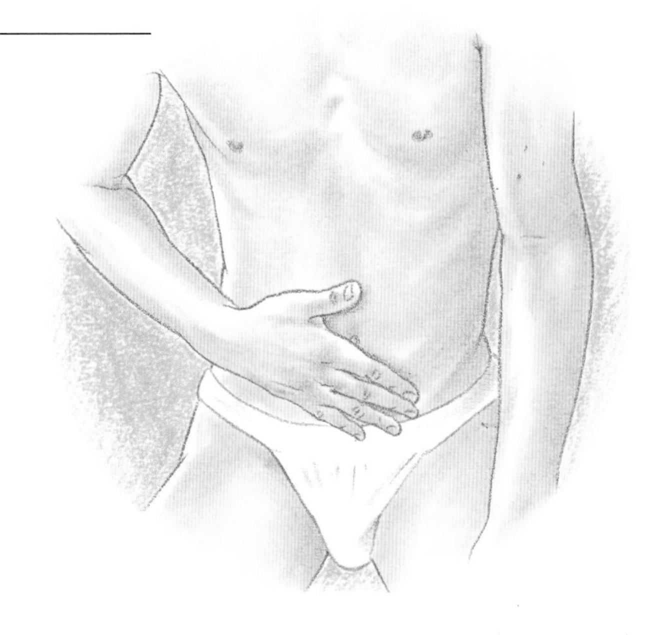

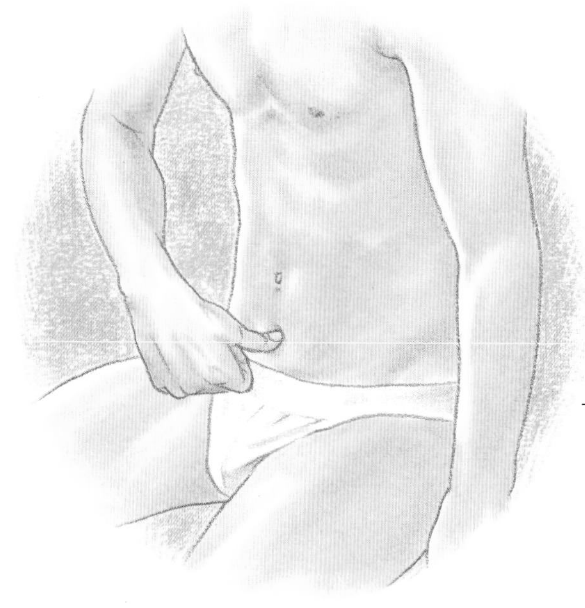

CAUTION
DO NOT PRACTISE MASSAGE IN THE ABDOMINAL REGION IF YOU ARE PREGNANT.

Kneading the lower abdomen

Located three inches (see pp. 32-3) below the navel on the midline of the belly is the acupoint Ren4 (*Guanyuan*). Knead Ren4 with your right thumb, applying a little more than moderate pressure. Repeat 50 to 100 times, alternating between clockwise and anticlockwise kneading.

Ren4 is a very important energy-giving acupoint (see p. 131). This massage is particularly beneficial when you are generally run down, or weak after illness and it also aids digestion. When applied to women, this massage helps to prevent menstrual problems.

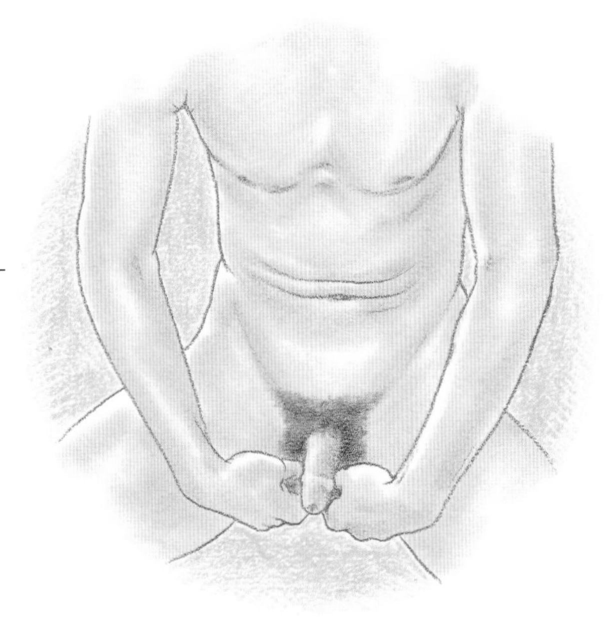

Squeezing the scrotum

Hold your scrotum in your hands, squeeze gently, and then release. Alternately squeeze and release in this way 50 times. If you prefer, you can do this massage through loose cotton underwear, such as boxer shorts.

This massage increases the production of male hormones, and maintains and promotes the healthy functioning of the male genitals. It also benefits the brain.

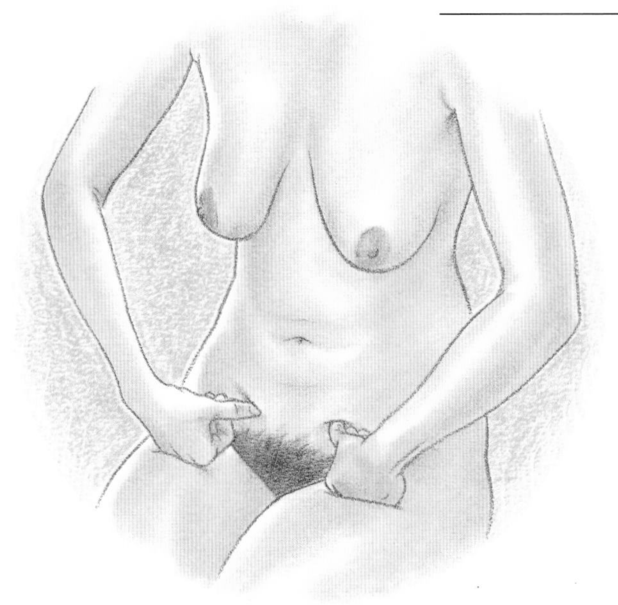

Kneading St29 ~ Guilai

This massage is for women only. With your thumbs, knead the points located 4 inches (see pp. 32-3) below the navel and 2 inches either side of the midline of the belly. This is the position of the St29 (*Guilai*) acupoints. Apply moderate pressure and make 50 small, circular kneading strokes.

St29 is an important acupoint for the reproductive organs (see p. 131). This kneading massage increases the production of female hormones, promotes the healthy functioning of the female reproductive organs, and also benefits the brain.

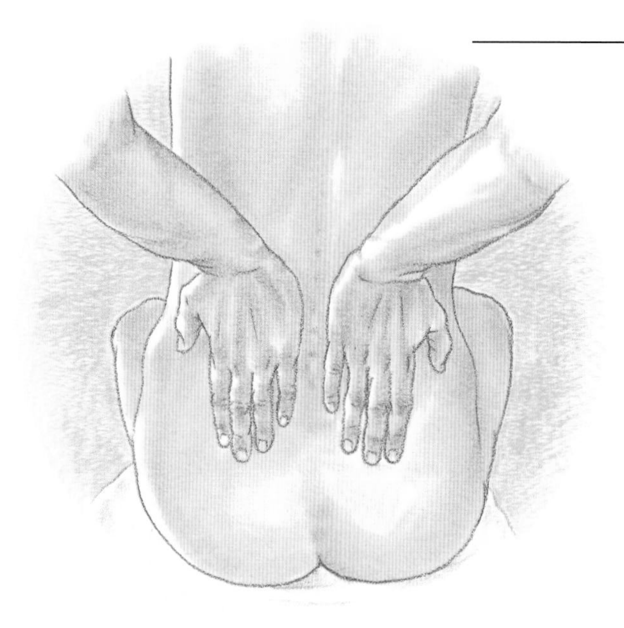

Rubbing the back

Rub your hands together, and when they are warm place them on your lower back 1.5 inches (see pp. 32-3) either side of the spine and level with the navel, on the acupoints UB23 (*Shenshu*). Rub the area with 50 to 100 fairly vigorous upward and downward strokes.

In Chinese medicine the Kidneys are regarded as fundamental organs, and UB23 (see p. 132) is the key acupoint related to the Kidneys. This massage maintains the healthy functioning of the Kidneys, and gives energy to the body. It also prevents insomnia, tinnitus, back pain, and diseases of the urogenital system.

CAUTION
DO NOT PRACTISE MASSAGE IN THE BACK REGION IF YOU ARE PREGNANT, OR DURING MENSTRUATION.

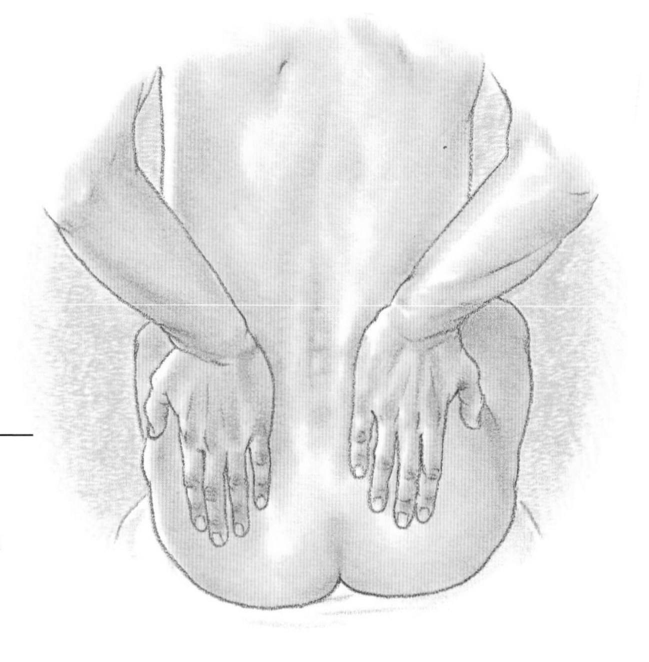

Rubbing the lower back

Warm your hands by rubbing them together. Then place them 4 inches (see pp. 32-3) from either side of your spine and level with the fourth lumbar vertebra. This is the location of the extra acupoints *Yoayan* (see p. 132). Rub up and down over the area fairly vigorously with your palms. Repeat 50 to 100 times.

This massage relieves back pain, and prevents kidney disease, insomnia, tinnitus, and diseases of the urogenital system.

SELF-CARE MASSAGE OF THE LIMBS

Rubbing the hands

Bring your hands together with your fingertips pointing upward. Keeping your shoulders relaxed, rub your palms together briskly 30 times.

The hand is the meeting place for the three Yin Hand Channels and the three Yang Hand Channels (see p. 10). This simple hand massage promotes the flexibility of the fingers and also benefits the brain and the Heart.

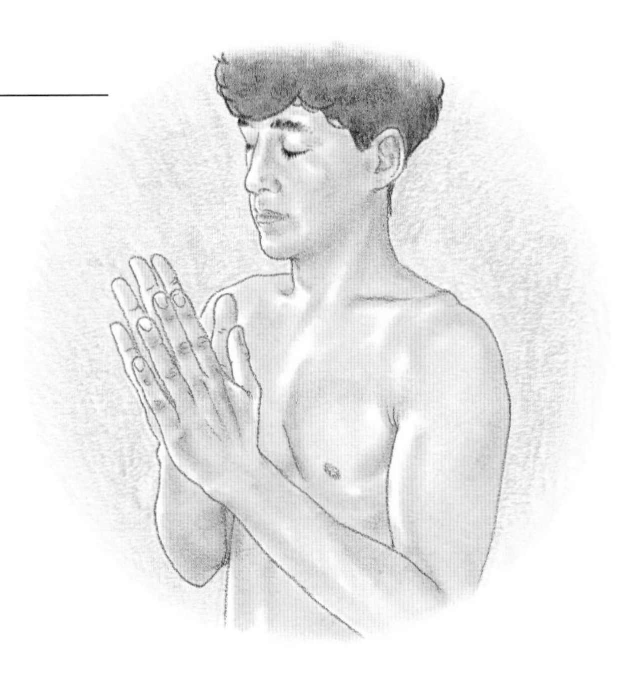

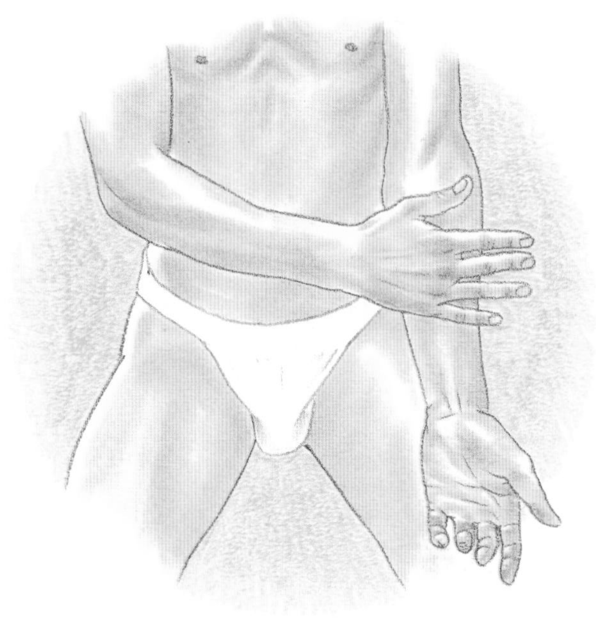

Rubbing the arms

Stretch your left arm in front of you, with your palm facing upward. With your right hand, rub your left arm from the wrist to just below the shoulder with a single, smooth, upward stroke. Turn your extended arm over so the palm is now facing downward. Then rub the arm in a downward direction to complete one sequence. Repeat the sequence 20 times on the left arm and then 20 times on the right arm.

This massage promotes Qi-blood flow in the arms. It also relieves arm pain and prevents digestive disorders.

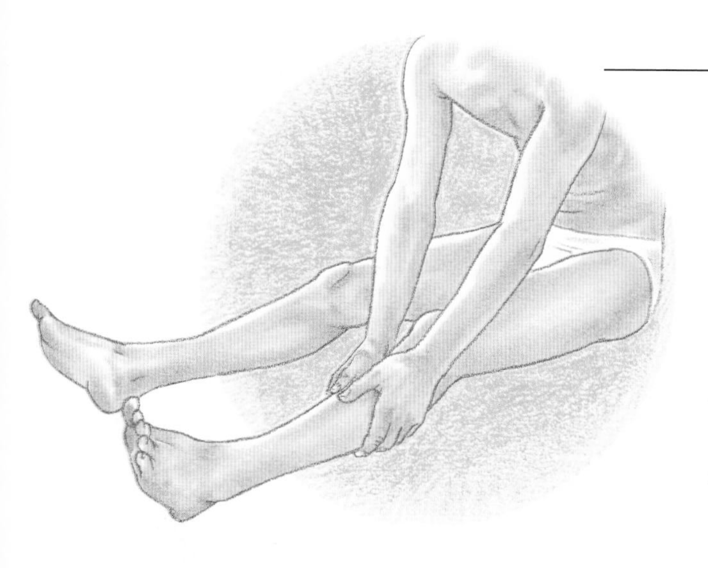

Rubbing the legs

Sit on the floor with your legs stretched out in front of you. Hold your left thigh with both hands and rub down the leg toward the ankle with some pressure. Then rub up the leg to complete one sequence. Repeat the sequence 20 times. Massage your right leg 20 times in the same way.

The leg contains the six Foot Channels. This massage relaxes the leg muscles, promotes the flow of blood in the leg, and improves the mobility of the leg.

Pressing the thighs

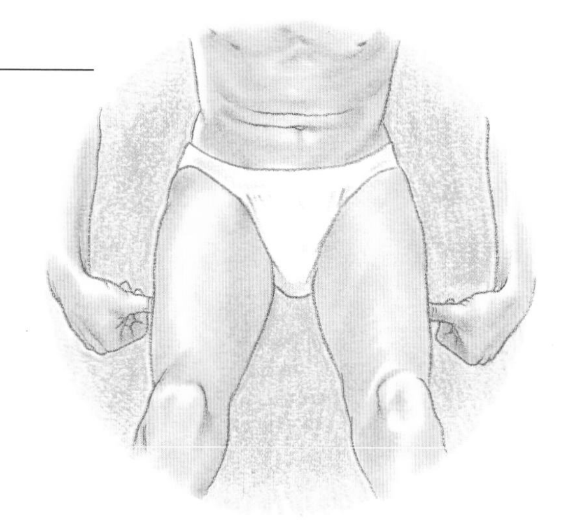

To locate the exact point to press, stand with your arms hanging down by your sides and mark the points that your middle fingers reach on each outer thigh. These are the GB31 (*Fengshi*) acupoints (see p. 137). Then sit on the floor with your legs stretched out in front of you and press GB31 on each thigh 30 times with your thumbs.

Apply this massage to relieve pain in the legs.

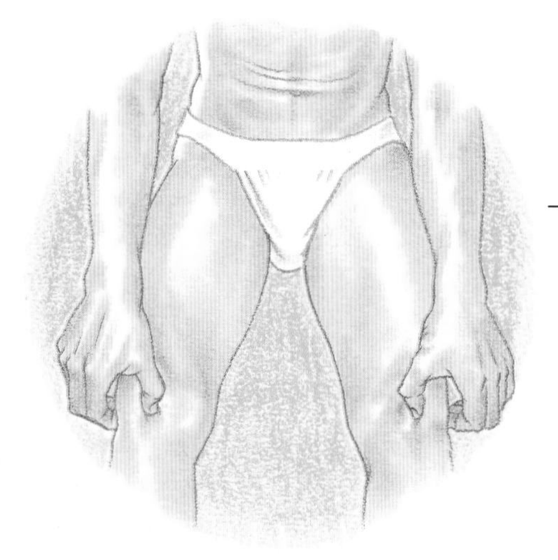

Kneading the knees

Sit on the floor with your legs stretched out in front of you. Find the two dimpled areas of each knee just below the kneecap. These are the two extra acupoints *Xiyan*. Knead these points in both knees with firm, circular strokes. Repeat 30 times.

Massage *Xiyan* (see p. 136) in this way to improve the mobility of the legs and prevent the onset of arthritis.

Pressing St36 ~ Zusanli

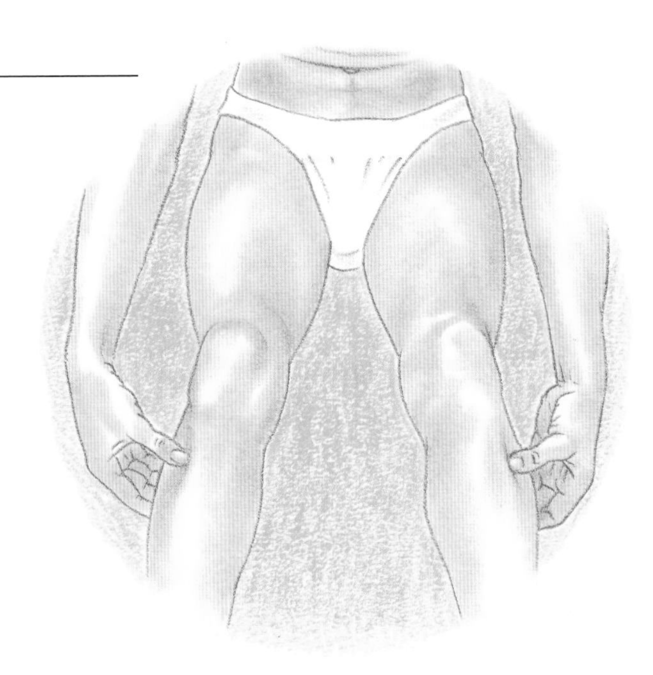

Sit with your legs stretched out in front of you. Find the St36 (*Zusanli*) acupoints 3 inches (see pp. 32-3) below the kneecap, on the outside of each tibia. Press acupoint St36 on each leg 30 times.

St36 is one of the energy-giving acupoints (see also p. 136). This massage promotes the circulation of blood in the legs and improves their motor function. It also improves your vitality and prevents diseases of the digestive system.

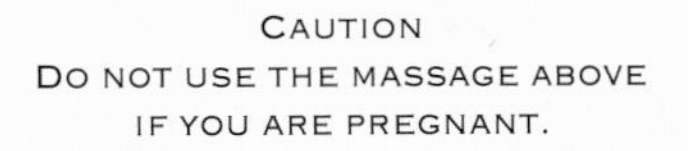

CAUTION
DO NOT USE THE MASSAGE ABOVE IF YOU ARE PREGNANT.

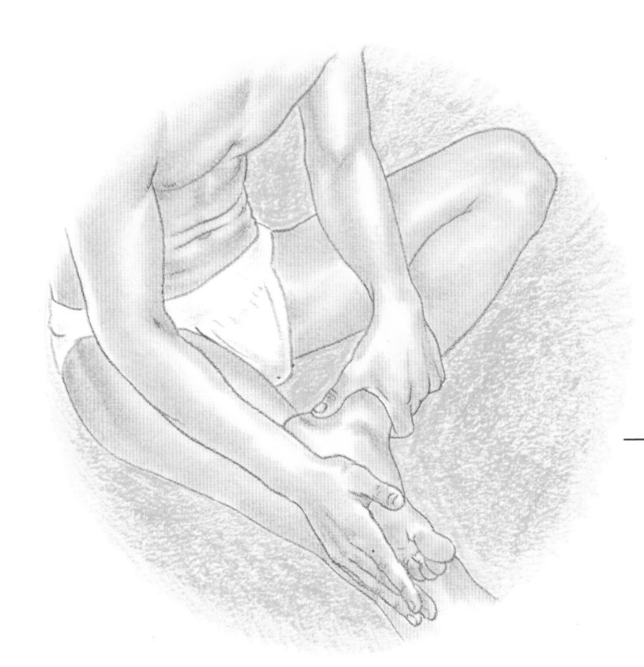

Rubbing the sole of the foot

Sit on the floor with your left leg bent in front of you. Rub your palms together until they are warm, then place your right palm on the sole of your left foot. Rub up and down over the area 30 times. Repeat the massage on the sole of your right foot.

Rubbing the foot improves the circulation, and prevents high blood pressure, anaemia, and insomnia. It also benefits the brain and the eyes.

CHAPTER TWO

LEARNING THE TECHNIQUES

CHINESE PAIN-RELIEF MASSAGE STOPS PAIN BY WORKING ON SPECIFIC ACUPOINTS, PAIN-RELIEF POINTS, AND CHANNELS AND ON THE AFFECTED PARTS OF THE BODY WITH MANIPULATIONS TO REMOVE QI-BLOOD STAGNATION, OPEN THE CHANNELS, AND BALANCE YIN AND YANG (SEE ALSO PP. 8-13), THUS RELIEVING PAIN.

CARE AND SENSITIVITY, A LITTLE TIME AND ENERGY, A WILLING PAIR OF HANDS, AND A KNOWLEDGE OF SOME BASIC MASSAGE MANIPULATIONS ARE ALL YOU NEED TO BEGIN. THIS CHAPTER COVERS THE FUNDAMENTALS OF PAIN-RELIEF MASSAGE, WITH GUIDELINES ON GENERALLY ACCEPTED PROCEDURES, AND DETAILED DESCRIPTIONS AND ILLUSTRATIONS OF THE COMMONLY USED MASSAGE STROKES AND TECHNIQUES. USE THIS CHAPTER AS A TEACHING AID TO HELP YOU TO LEARN THE BASICS, AND AS A SOURCE OF REFERENCE WHEN YOU ARE FOLLOWING THE TREATMENT INSTRUCTIONS IN THE REST OF THE BOOK.

REMEMBER, THE EFFECTIVENESS OF PAIN-RELIEF MASSAGE DEPENDS ON THE QUALITY OF THE MANIPULATION. AS A BEGINNER, DON'T BE DAUNTED BY HOW MUCH THERE IS TO LEARN. PERSEVERE, AND YOU WILL COME TO UNDERSTAND THE TECHNIQUES AND APPLY THEM WITH SUCCESS.

Procedure for treatment

Pain-relief massage is usually performed using one of two broad methods. The effects of each are quite different. The first technique is to massage in a centrifugal direction, that is, away from the heart. Centrifugal massage promotes healthy blood circulation and increases the metabolism. The second method is centripetal massage, which is directed toward the heart. Centripetal massage speeds up the return of blood and lymph. It also helps to reduce swelling and dispel Qi-blood stagnation.

Your strokes

The manipulations are for specific movements and will require practice. Try the strokes out on your own body while sitting or lying on the floor or in bed. With practice you will find that your hands relax and the manipulations begin to come naturally to you.

Your massage strokes should be even and reasonably forceful, so that they are deep and thorough. Your movements should always be continuous, elastic and, above all, rhythmic. Your hands and arms should be relaxed as you perform the strokes.

Effective pain-relief massage relies on the correct choice of manipulation and the correct implementation of the technique. With experience you will choose appropriate massage strokes to treat various types of pain, and will improve your techniques. Not only will your strokes improve, but also your understanding, and your ability to apply the principles of duration, repetition, and pressure in a flexible way.

Strength of massage

You can practise most of the manipulations in this chapter either gently, moderately, or with intense pressure. However, "gentle" does not mean without any force at all, and "intense" does not imply either roughness or hardness. Vary the pressure, speed, and frequency of your hand actions according to each case. In general, use slower and gentler actions to treat thinner, weaker people, and those suffering from chronic, debilitating diseases. When treating strong, young, or well-built people, use quicker movements and apply more intense pressure.

As a rule, the manipulations should be gentle at the beginning and toward the end of a sequence, and stronger in the middle. For example, at the beginning of a massage session you could use rubbing (MO), pushing (TUI), or rotatory kneading (ROU), practising them all fairly gently. Then, for the main treatment use other manipulations, such as pressing (AN), rotatory kneading (ROU), squeezing (NA), and pinching (QIA), which you should perform more firmly. Toward the end of the sequence, be gentle again; and where appropriate, include massage techniques such as circling (YAO), light percussing (KOU), and gentle tapping (PAI).

The routine

When giving a full body-massage, ideally you should start at the head and then go on to massage the rest of the body – the chest and stomach, the back, then the arms, and finally the legs. However, this sequence is not fixed and you can change it according to each individual case. As far as possible, try to move your partner as little as possible during treatment.

Course of treatment

In general, a course of treatment comprises ten massage sessions. The frequency of these sessions depends on your partner's symptoms. Treat someone suffering from acute pain with pain-relief massage every day or at least every other day. Massage those with more chronic symptoms two to four times per week.

A massage session usually lasts about half an hour. You may need about one hour if the whole body is treated.

Before you start

You can give massage for pain relief almost anywhere. A therapist may use a consulting room, but you can use any room at home or even in the office. You do not need any particular space or equipment; however, the more you can do to create a calm and comfortable setting, the more

Hot compresses

A hot compress is sometimes suggested after massage to improve the local circulation of blood and to relieve pain further. To prepare a hot compress soak a towel or flannel in hot water (50°C), and then apply it to the affected part of the body. Replace the compress with a new, hot one as soon as the original compress has cooled to luke warm. You should apply a hot compress to the affected area for 15 to 20 minutes every evening until the condition has improved.

effective your treatment will be, since relaxation is central to any form of massage.

You can practise pain-relief massage without any accompaniments or, in some instances, you can apply surgical spirits to the skin to improve the effect of the massage. The surgical spirits help to relax the muscles and tendons, improve Qi flow, and dispel Cold and Damp (see p. 9). Have a bottle of surgical spirits ready before you start a massage session.

Some of the treatments in Chapter Four, Relieving Pain, suggest that you apply a hot compress to the affected part after massage (see the box on the facing page). A hot compress helps to relieve pain further, and improves the local circulation of blood.

Reactions to treatment

Your partner should feel relaxed and comfortable after massage. Occasionally an individual may feel uncomfortable or experience more pain in the affected part, particularly after their first few sessions. Allow someone new to pain-relief massage time to become familiar with the techniques by using moderate pressures and speeds for their initial sessions.

Experiencing some soreness and pain in the acupoints after massage is normal and it should soon pass. However, take care not to apply too much force and avoid excessively hard and rough hand actions that may damage your partner's skin. Be very gentle when treating the old and those with osteoporosis.

Pay constant attention to your partner's reaction to treatment. In time, you will learn to adjust the pressure, speed, and frequency of the manipulations to the limit of an individual's endurance, and to suit your partner's case.

Practitioner's checklist

- Make the massage room as warm, inviting, and quiet as possible. Keep the temperature at a constant level.

- Your partner can either lie on a massage table, or on any other long sturdy table, in bed, or on blankets on the floor. For some treatments, sitting in a chair may be appropriate. The important thing is that your partner is comfortable.

- Before you begin a massage, wash your hands and check that your fingernails are short. Take off your watch and any rings or bracelets, and ask your partner to do the same.

- Encourage your partner to relax completely before and during treatment. Check that he or she has visited the toilet before you start.

- Your partner can be either naked or clothed during the massage, as long as the area being treated is bare for massage. Always respect your partner's need for privacy.

- Choose a comfortable position from which to practise the massage, and ensure that you can reach the required acupoints easily. If you feel slightly awkward you may not be able to exert pressure effectively.

- Always wash your hands at the end of a massage session.

Methods of locating acupoints

Throughout this book you will need to be able to locate specific acupoints accurately. The location of an acupoint is commonly described in terms of the number of inches from a body landmark. For example, in the Appendix, Ren14 (*Juque*) is described as being 6 inches above the navel, on the midline of the belly. However, the "inch" unit referred to differs from the imperial inch measurement, as the exact length of the inch unit applied in Chinese massage is unique to each individual. The method of using body landmarks to find an acupoint is described here, as well as two methods using Chinese anatomical inch units to locate acupoints – finger measure and bone-length measure.

You can use just one of these methods, but in practice a combination of all three methods is most effective. With experience you will recognize when you have found the precise point. A useful guide is that the correct point may feel sore and painful when pressed.

Body landmarks

Obvious anatomical features such as the eyebrows, navel, and nipples, are used as landmarks for locating acupoints. For example, the extra acupoint *Yintang* is located midway between the eyebrows, and Ren17 (*Tanzhong*) lies midway between the nipples. Other landmarks commonly referred to include the hairlines, various bones, creases in the skin for example at the elbow, wrist, and knee, and the spinal vertebrae. Refer to the Body Landmarks map (see p. 140) to help you to locate any bones and anatomical features that you are unfamiliar with.

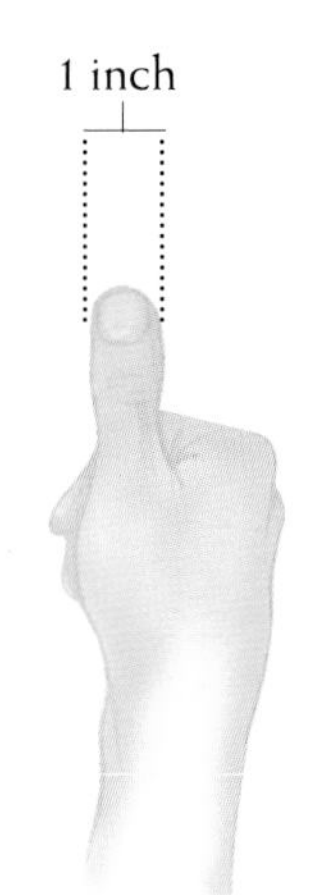

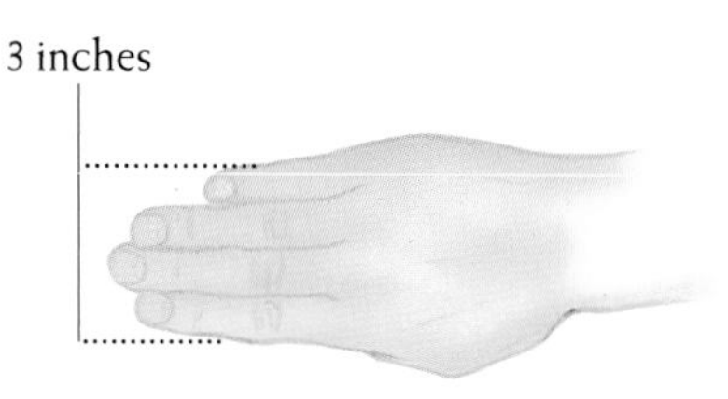

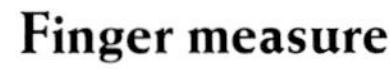

Finger measure

This method uses the width of a person's own fingers as a unit of measurement. For example, the width of the thumb is taken as one "inch", and the combined width of the index and middle finger is taken as 1.5 inches. If you have a similar frame to your partner, you can use your own fingers as a guide to locating acupoints. This measure is easy to use, but perhaps less precise than the bone-length measure method (see p. 33).

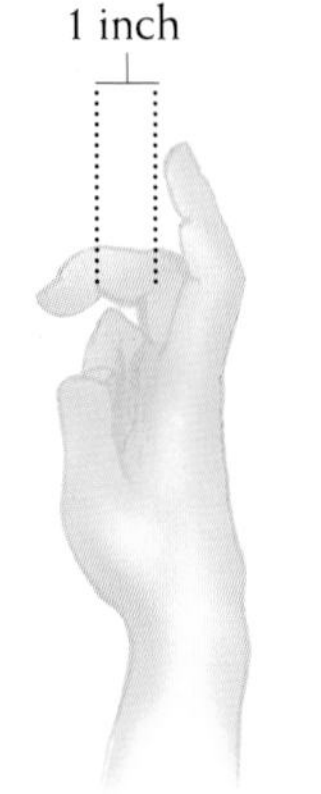

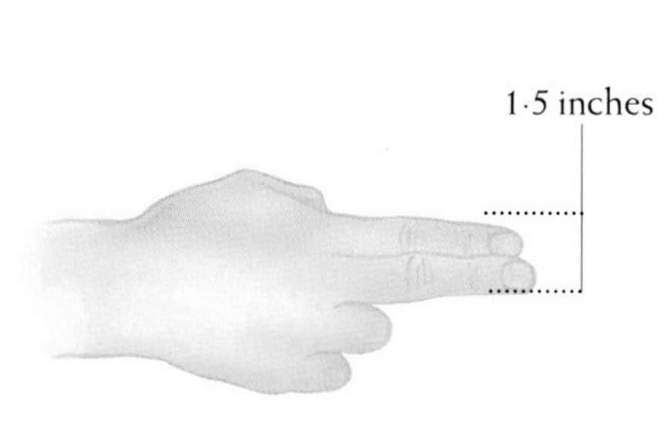

Bone-length measure

This method of locating acupoints divides up parts of the body into a set number of units of equal length. For example, the distance between the armpit crease and the elbow crease is divided into 9 equal units, and the distance between the elbow crease and the wrist crease is said to be 12 equal units (see below). In Chinese massage each unit is said to be one inch. The number of inches between each section of the body is the same for each individual, but the actual length of the inch varies according to the frame of the individual.

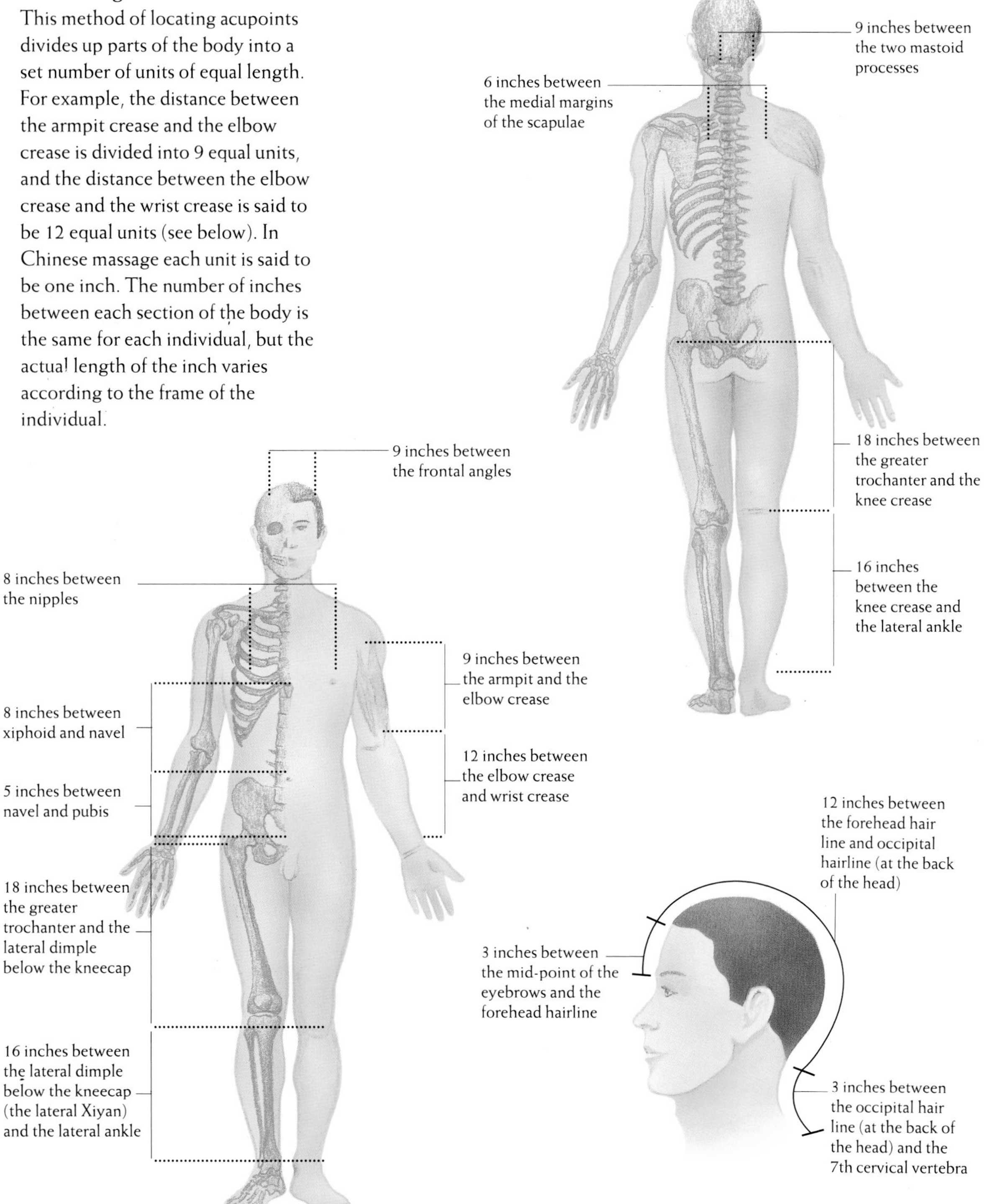

PRESSING ~ *AN*

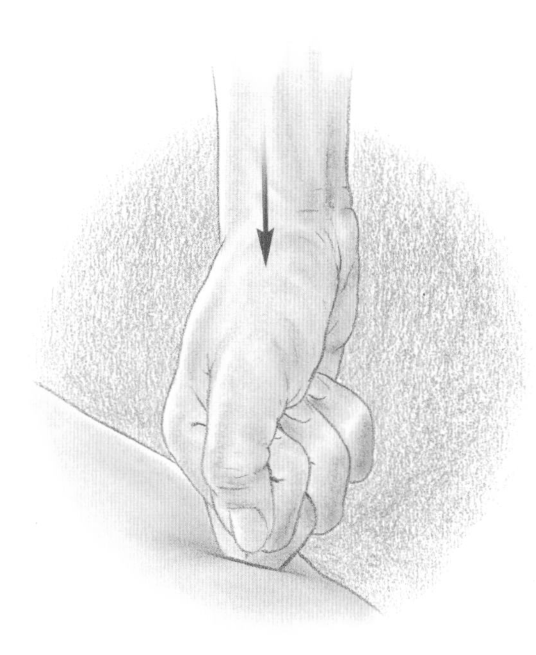

AN with the knuckle

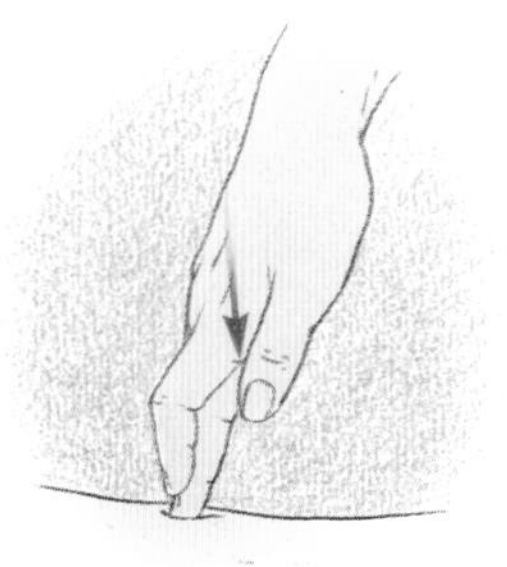

AN with the middle finger

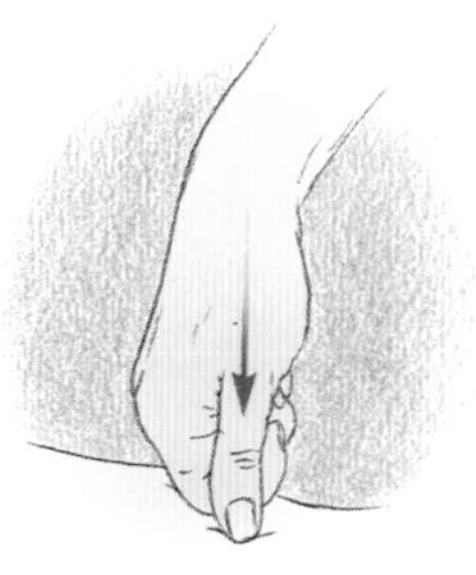

AN with the thumb

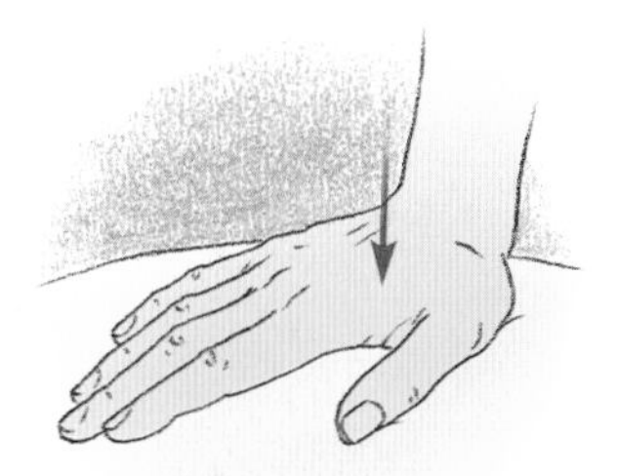

AN with the palm

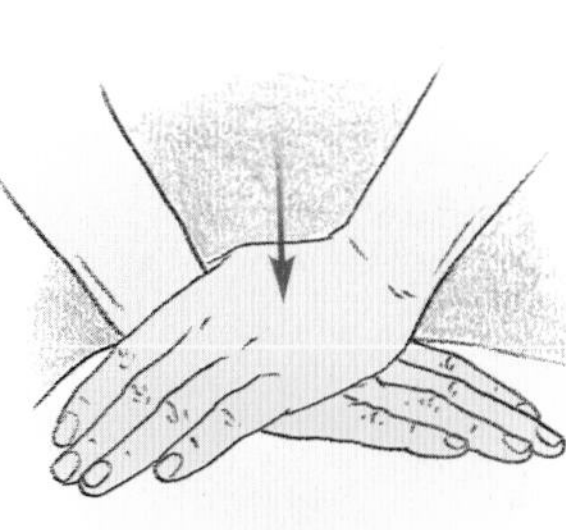

AN with the palms

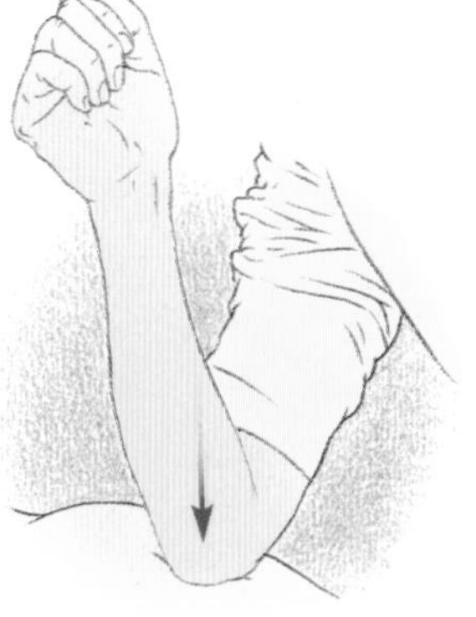

AN with the elbow

AN is the Chinese term for applying pressure to an acupoint or part of the body by pressing. Use your finger or knuckle to press an acupoint, and use your palm or elbow to press more muscular parts of the body, such as the chest, abdomen, back, and buttocks.

You can apply AN in two ways. Either begin by pressing gently and gradually press harder until the patient feels quite an intense pressure – a feeling that should last only for a moment. Alternatively, apply continuous, moderate pressure using rhythmic and elastic movements. Take care not to damage the skin by pressing either too roughly or too hard.

USE AN TO CLEAR THE CHANNELS, TO DISPERSE STAGNATED QI AND BLOOD, AND TO ALLEVIATE PAIN.

PUSHING ~ *TUI*

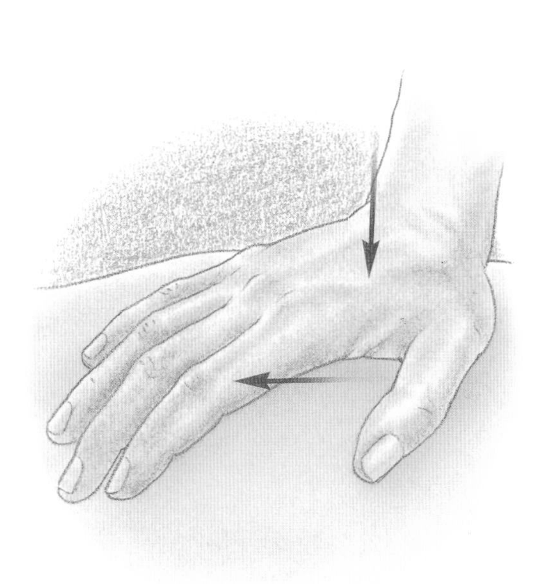

Tui with the palm

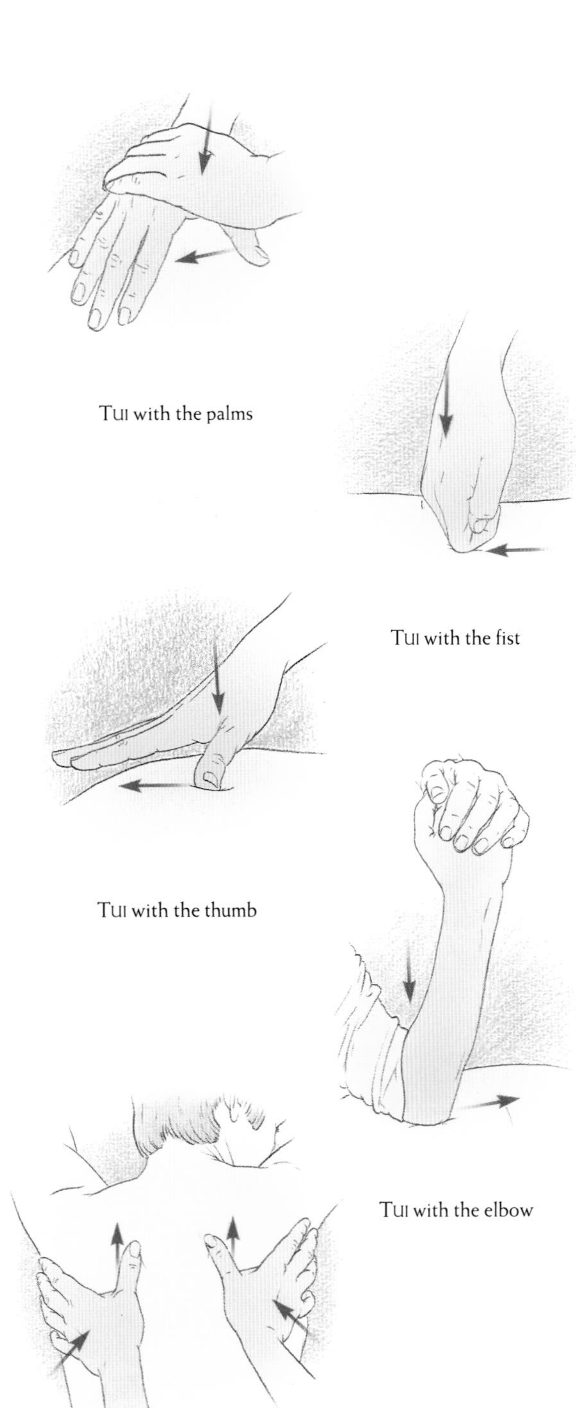

Tui with the palms

Tui with the fist

Tui with the thumb

Tui with the elbow

Tui applied to the back

Tui is the Chinese term for the pushing massage technique. Apply a moderate amount of pressure as you push the selected massage "tool" in one direction over the skin. Gently return your hand to the start point and repeat the pushing stroke.

You can apply Tui anywhere on the body if you select the appropriate "tool". Use the fist or the elbow on muscular areas, and either the thumb or the heel of the hand on more sensitive areas such as the face. Vary the pressure and speed of the massage according to the health of your partner and the condition of the affected part. Take particular care when treating swollen areas.

TUI RELAXES THE MUSCLES AND TENDONS, RELIEVES SPASM AND PAIN, PROMOTES BLOOD CIRCULATION, INCREASES THE SKIN'S ELASTICITY, AND HELPS TO OVERCOME FATIGUE.

RUBBING ~ *MO*

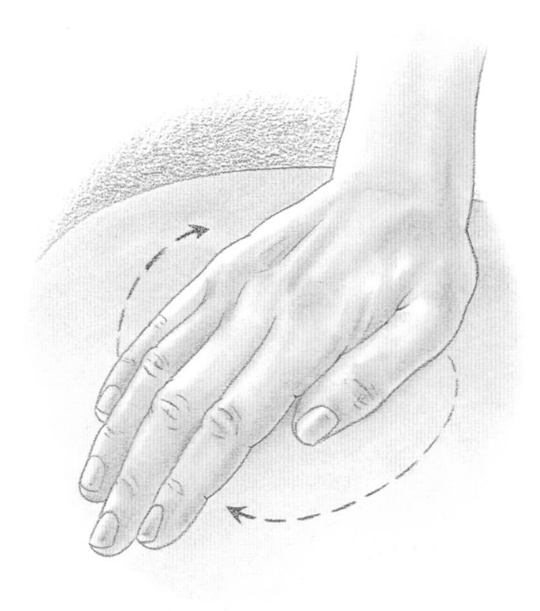

Mo with the palm

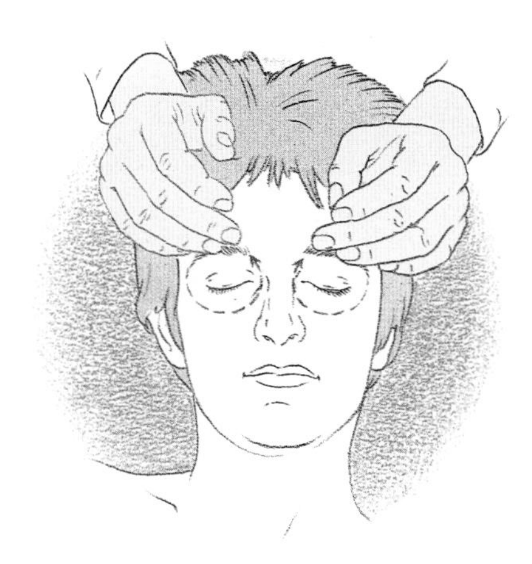

Mo applied around the eyes

Mo is the Chinese massage term for rubbing the body. Place either the fingers or palm on the required acupoint or treatment area and rub the skin using circular strokes. You can either apply Mo to a specific area with small, circular rubbing movements, or use more sweeping, broader strokes to massage over a larger area. In all cases, apply smooth, constant pressure, to penetrate the subcutaneous layer, but no deeper. Apply Mo to the back, abdomen, soles of the feet, and around the eyes.

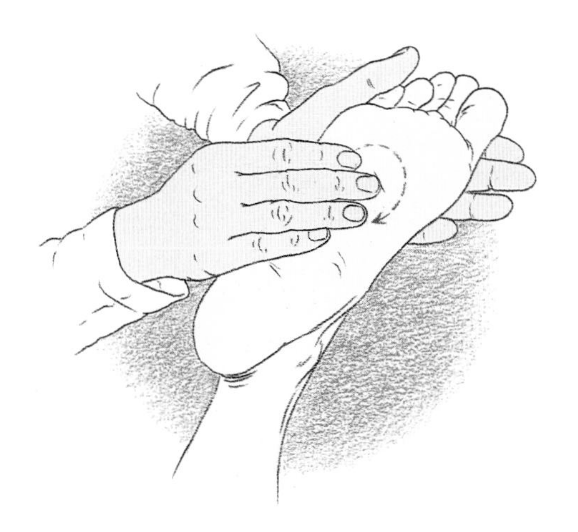

Mo with the fingers

USE MO TO REGULATE QI-BLOOD FLOW, TO REDUCE SWELLING AND PAIN, TO STRENGTHEN THE SPLEEN AND STOMACH AND THE OTHER VISCERA (SEE P. 9), AND TO INCREASE THE ELASTICITY OF THE SKIN.

KNEADING ~ *ROU*

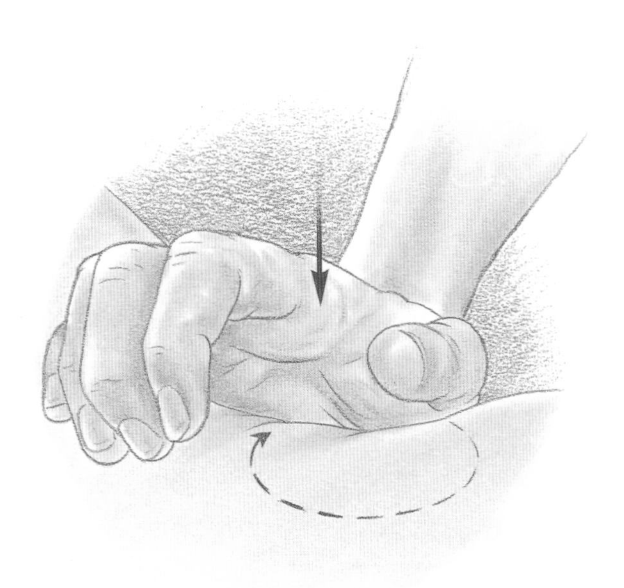

ROU with the heel of the hand

ROU is the Chinese rotatory kneading massage technique. It involves exerting a firm, even, and steady pressure in a circular manner. Use either your finger, palm, heel of the palm, thenar (the side of the thumb), thumb, or elbow to knead the required acupoint or affected area. First knead in a clockwise circle and then in an anticlockwise direction. Gradually increase the pressure applied and then reduce it again. ROU is a moderately firm stroke, which can be applied to all parts of the body. It is often used with AN, the pressing manipulation (see p. 34).

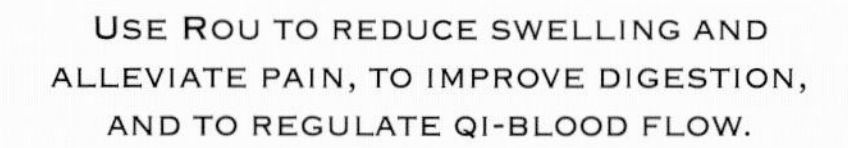

USE ROU TO REDUCE SWELLING AND ALLEVIATE PAIN, TO IMPROVE DIGESTION, AND TO REGULATE QI-BLOOD FLOW.

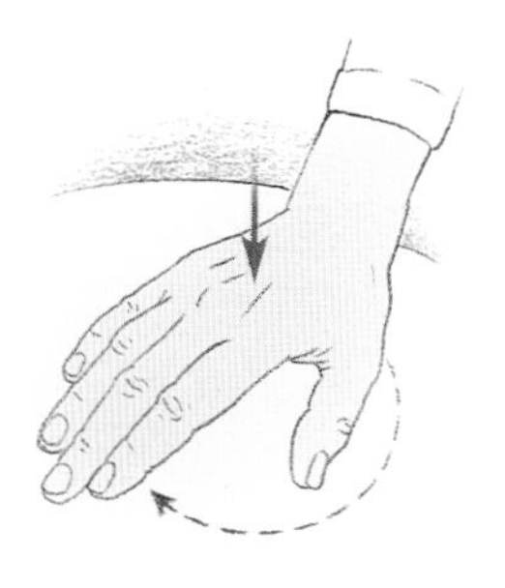

ROU with the palm

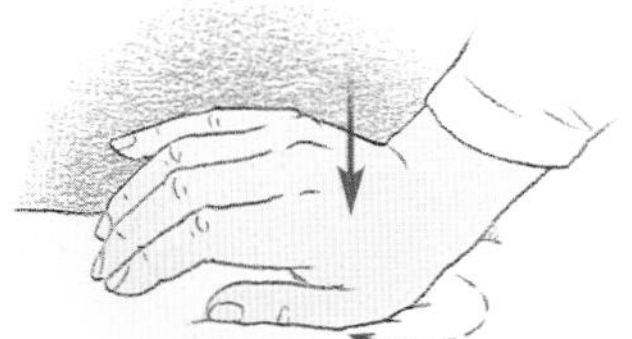

ROU with the thenar

ROU with the palms

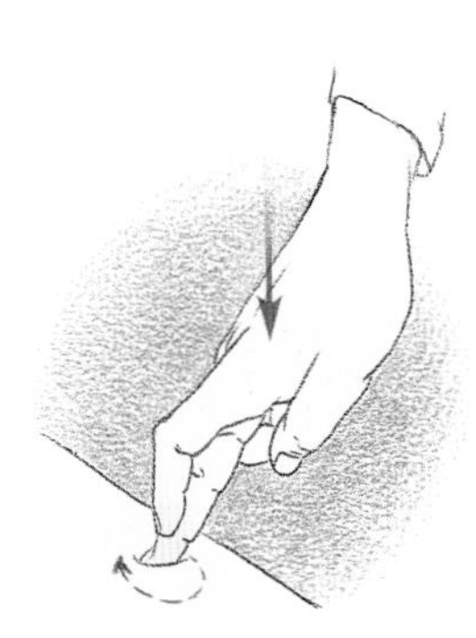

ROU with the middle finger

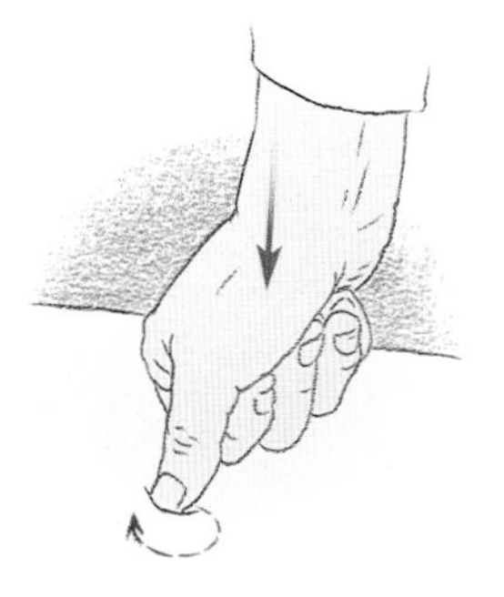

ROU with the thumb

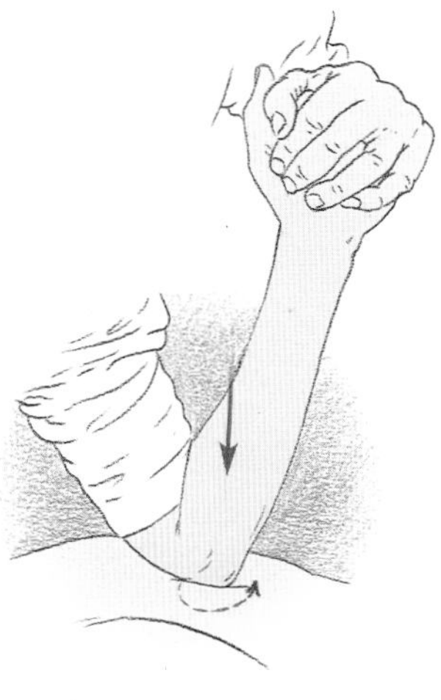

ROU with the elbow

PINCHING ~ *QIA*

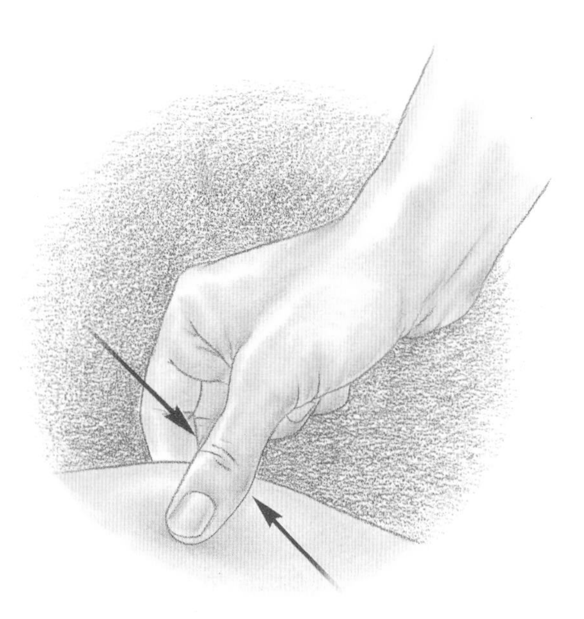

QIA with the fingers

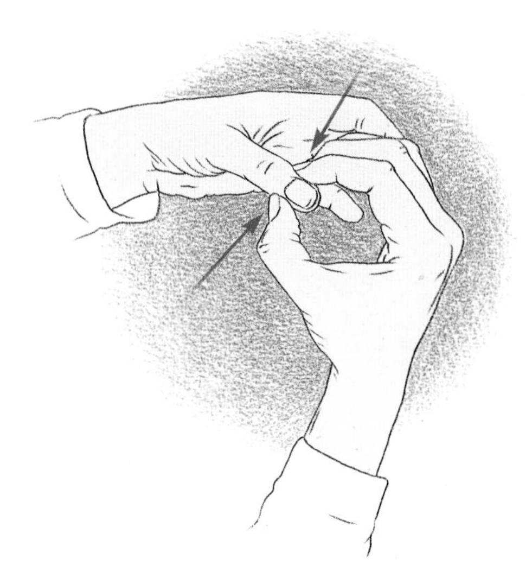

QIA applied to the finger

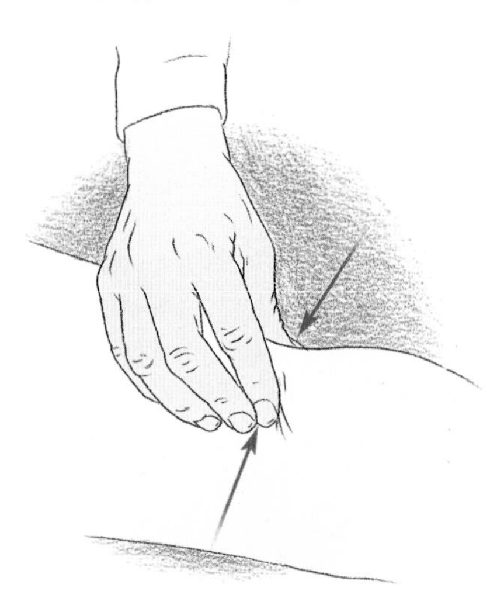

QIA applied to the leg

QIA is the Chinese term for pinching. Pinch the required acupoint or treatment area between the tip of your thumb and the tips of your index and middle fingers. Pinch firmly and hold with continuous, forceful pressure. QIA is an intense manipulation. Your partner will feel sore and experience some pain as you pinch, but this should soon subside. However, take care not to exceed your partner's pain threshold, or to damage the skin.

USE QIA TO STIMULATE ACUPOINTS, TO CLEAR THE CHANNELS, AND TO REDUCE THE SWELLING OF SOFT TISSUES.

SQUEEZING ~ *NA*

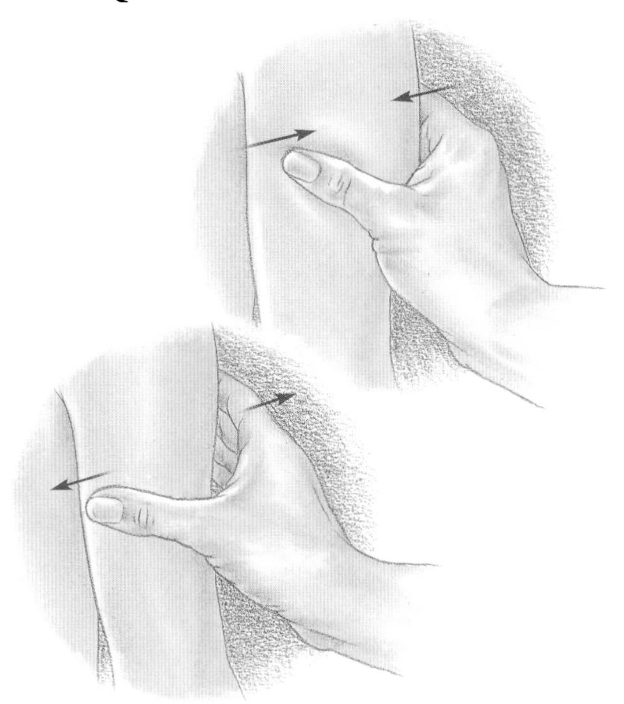

NA applied to the arm

NA is the Chinese term for the squeezing massage technique. You can apply NA to most parts of the body, such as the limbs, the neck and shoulders, and the back. Adopt a pincer-like position with your hand using your thumb either with your index and middle finger, or with all your fingers. Repeatedly squeeze and release the acupoint or the required part of the body. Keep your wrist relaxed, and your squeezing action slow and rhythmical. During the course of this massage, gradually increase the force you apply and then reduce it again.

NA RELIEVES MUSCULAR SPASM, AND REGULATES NERVE FUNCTION. APPLY NA TO UNBLOCK THE CHANNELS, TO OVERCOME FATIGUE, AND TO DISPEL COLD (SEE P. 9).

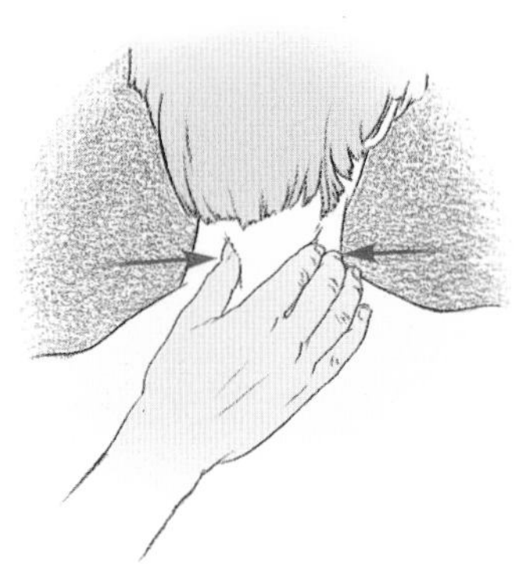

NA applied to the neck

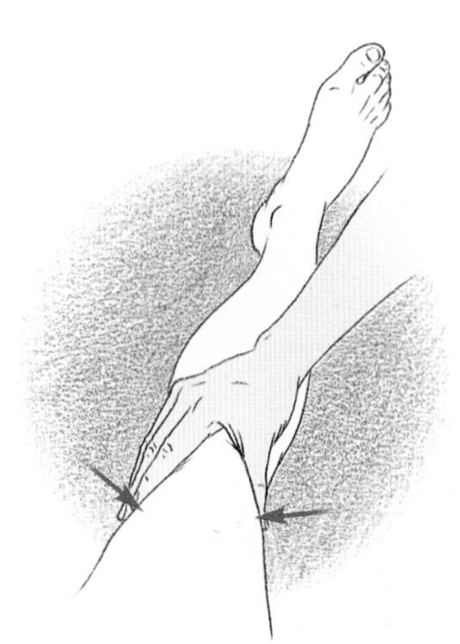

NA applied to the leg

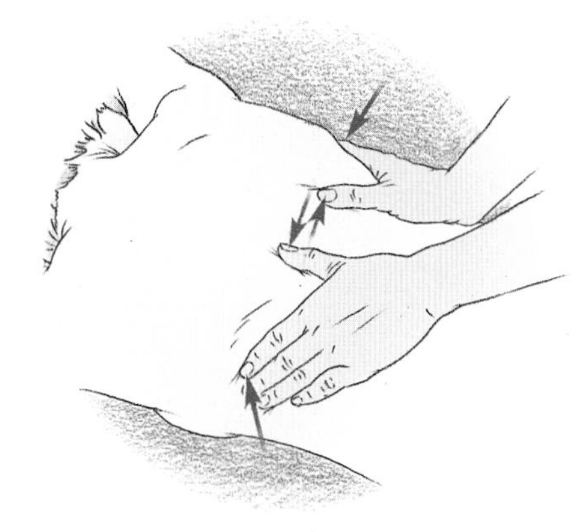

NA applied to the back

WIPING ~ *MO2*

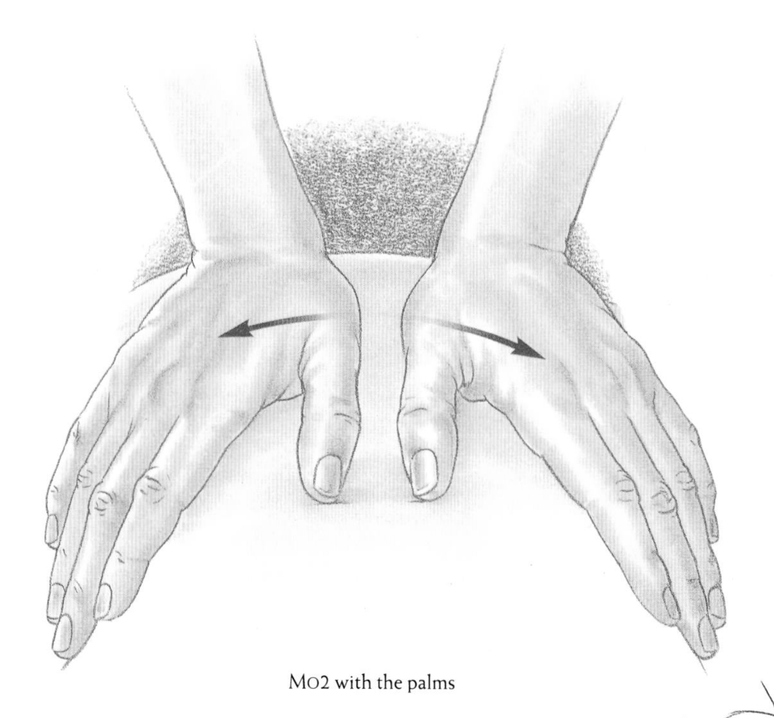

MO2 with the palms

Although it has the same pronunciation as the third manipulation, this MO refers to a different massage technique. To avoid confusion we will call it MO2. It involves pushing your hands or thumbs apart in opposite directions from a central point. Gently place both thumbs or palms side by side, on the required part of the body, and push them apart slowly with fluent and moderate strokes. Apply even and equal pressure with both hands. This soothing technique is usually applied to the forehead, neck, back, and abdomen.

MO2 applied to the back

MO2 IS A CALMING MASSAGE STROKE. USE IT TO REDUCE OVER-EXCITEMENT. MO2 IS ALSO VERY INVIGORATING, AND INCREASES THE ELASTICITY OF THE SKIN.

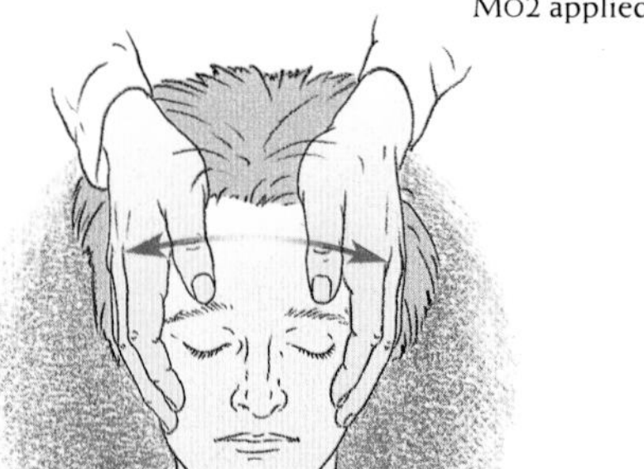

MO2 applied to the forehead

ROLLING ~ *GUN*

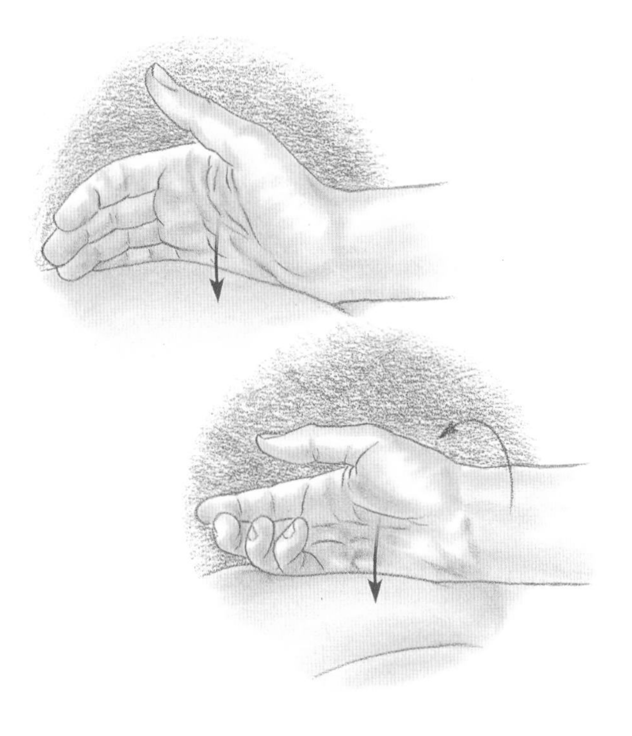

GUN is the Chinese rolling massage technique. It is used to treat muscular parts of the body. Place the outer side of your hand on the required part of the body. Your hand should be relaxed and your fingers slightly curled. Roll your hand to and fro in a rhythmic and even manner, and apply enough pressure to penetrate the muscle layer.

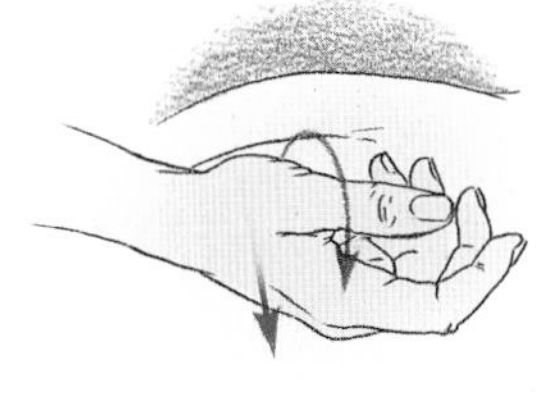

USE GUN TO RELAX THE MUSCLES AND TENDONS, TO RELIEVE MUSCULAR SPASMS, PAIN, AND FATIGUE, TO STRENGTHEN THE BONES, AND TO EASE JOINT MOVEMENT. IT ALSO IMPROVES BLOOD CIRCULATION.

QUIVERING ~ *ZHEN*

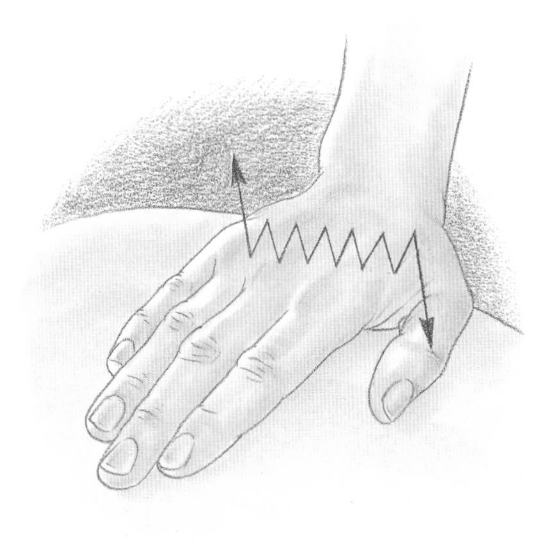

ZHEN with the palm

The quivering massage technique is known as ZHEN in Chinese massage. Apply intense pressure to the required part of the body using your fingertips or one or both palms, and make a rapid, continuous, quivering action. Apply firm pressure to penetrate deep down through the skin.

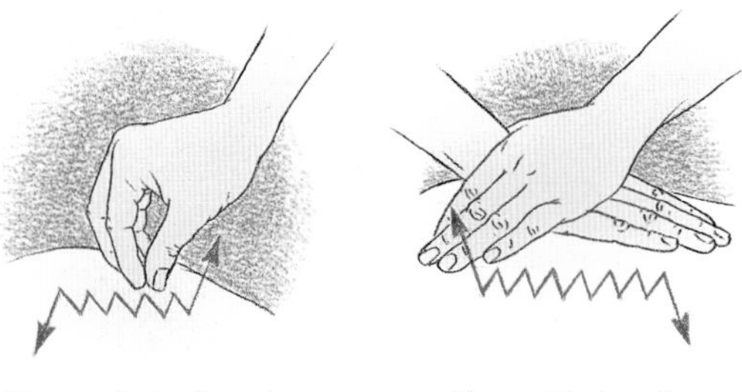

ZHEN with the fingertips

ZHEN with the palms

USE ZHEN TO RELAX THE MUSCLES, AND TO RELIEVE MUSCULAR SPASMS AND PAIN. IT ALSO HELPS TO OVERCOME FATIGUE.

TAPPING ~ *PAI*

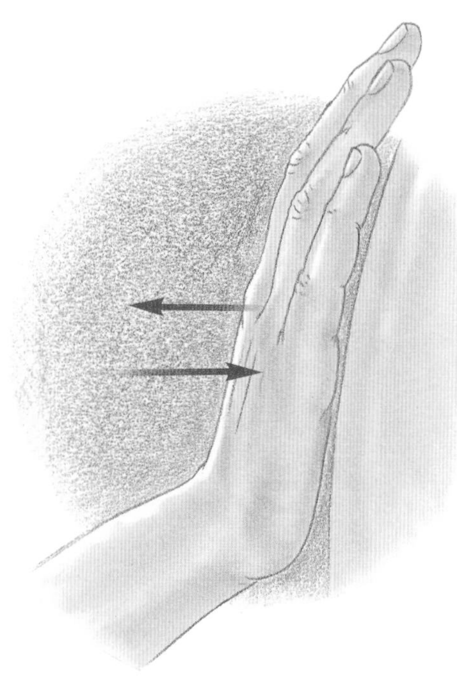

Pai with the palm

Pai is the Chinese term for the tapping massage technique. Use your palm, the back of your hand, or your fingertips to tap the required part of the body. Keep your wrist relaxed, and the tapping action gentle, even, elastic, and rhythmic. Pai is a much gentler technique than Kou (see facing page), with which it is often used. Use Pai toward the end of a massage sequence.

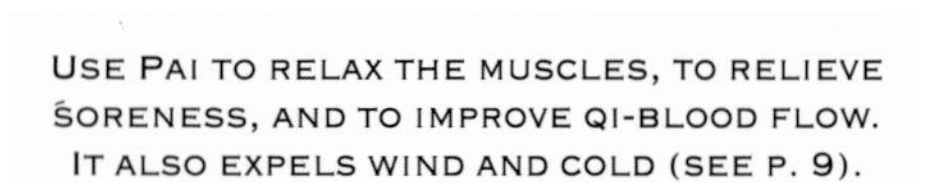

USE PAI TO RELAX THE MUSCLES, TO RELIEVE SORENESS, AND TO IMPROVE QI-BLOOD FLOW. IT ALSO EXPELS WIND AND COLD (SEE P. 9).

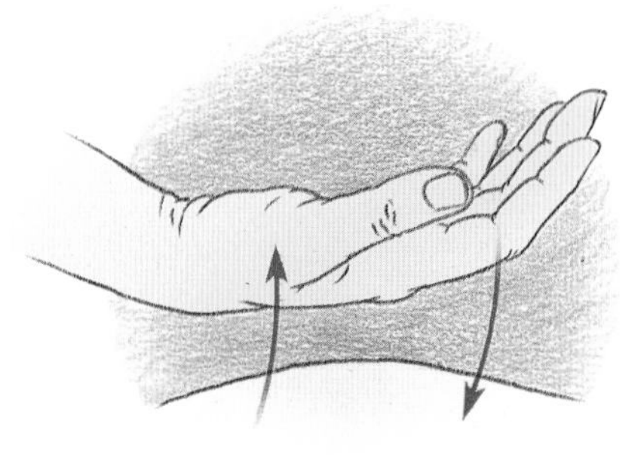

Pai with the back of the hand

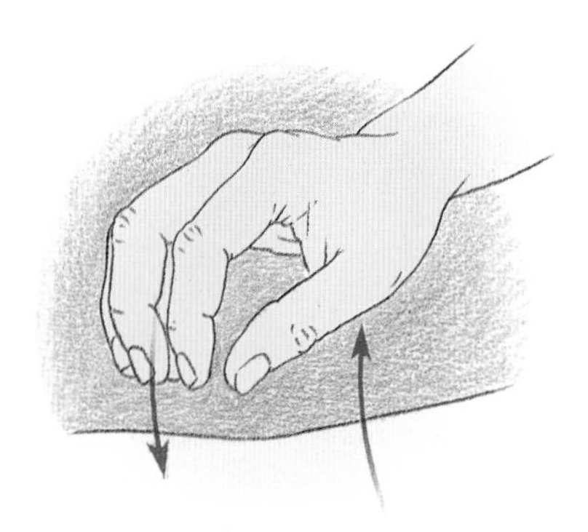

Pai with the tips of the fingers

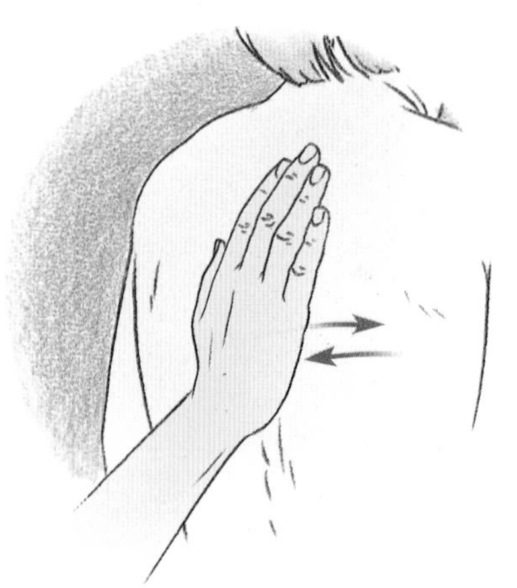

Pai applied to the back

PERCUSSING ~ *KOU*

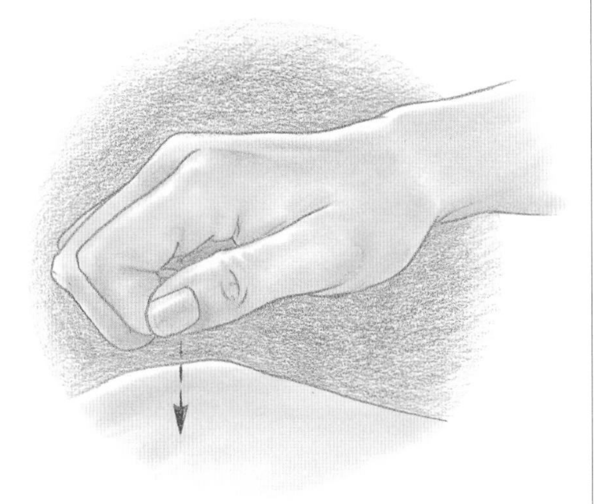

Kou with the fist

Kou is the Chinese percussing manipulation. Clench your fist loosely and use the flattened finger surface (but not the knuckles) to percuss the required point or part of the body. You can also use your fingertips for this manipulation. Keep your wrist relaxed and flexible, and the percussing action rhythmic and elastic. Apply Kou to the legs, shoulders, and back.

APPLY KOU TO IMPROVE QI-BLOOD FLOW, TO RELAX THE MUSCLES, AND TO HELP OVERCOME FATIGUE.

TWISTING ~ *CUO*

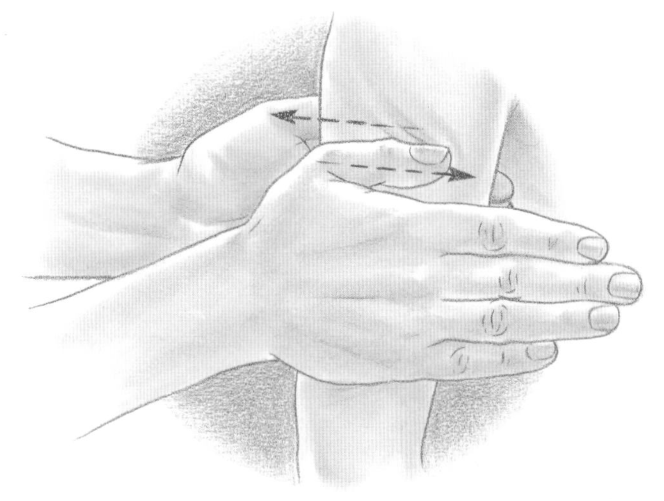

Cuo applied to the arm

Cuo is the Chinese twisting massage technique, which is used on the arms and legs. Hold the required limb firmly between your palms and move your hands back and forth in a rhythmical, alternating way, as if you are twisting a rope. Increase the speed of Cuo gradually during the course of the massage and then reduce it.

USE CUO TO UNBLOCK THE CHANNELS AND TO REGULATE QI-BLOOD FLOW. CUO EASES JOINT MOVEMENT, RELAXES THE MUSCLES, AND HELPS TO OVERCOME FATIGUE.

SHAKING ~ *DOU*

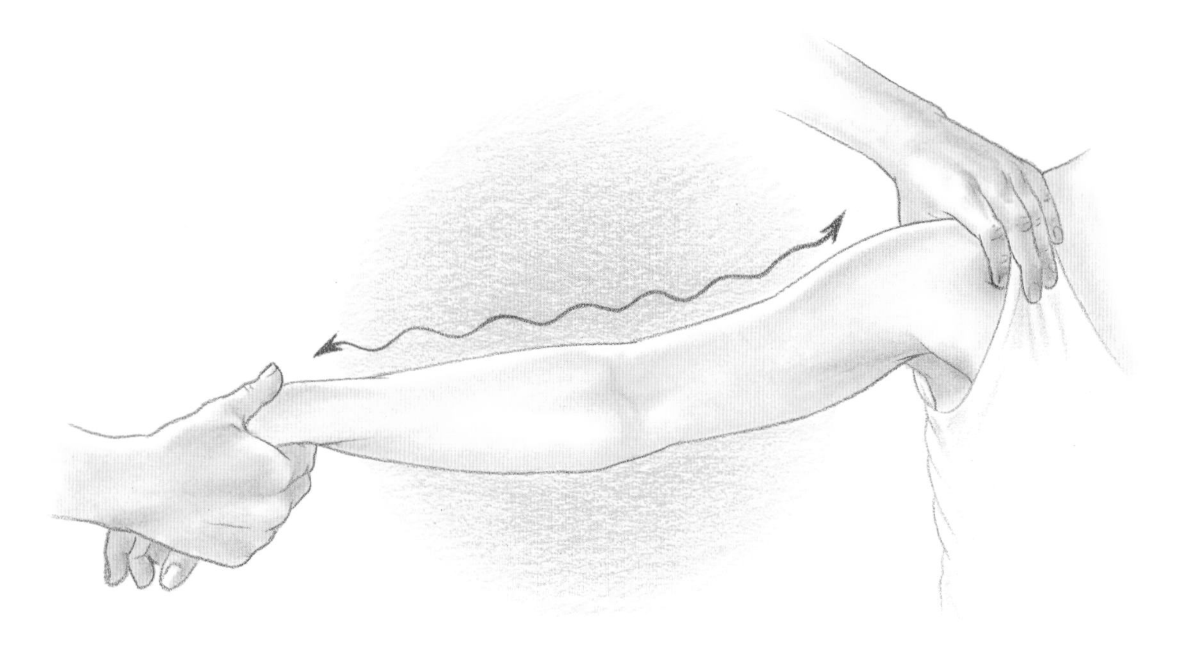

Dou applied to the arm

Dou is the Chinese massage technique that involves shaking your partner's arms or legs. Ask your partner to relax the affected limb, then hold it firmly and shake it up and down as if it were a rope. The range of movement is narrow; only move the limb up and down, and do not let it twist. You can gradually increase the speed of shaking, but it should never be too quick. Dou is usually applied with Yao (see facing page).

Dou applied to the legs

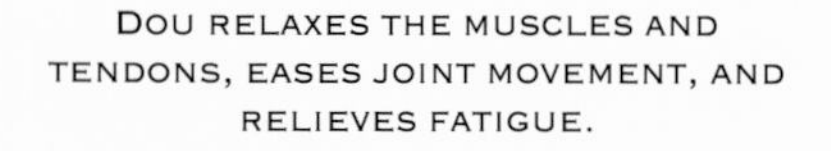

DOU RELAXES THE MUSCLES AND TENDONS, EASES JOINT MOVEMENT, AND RELIEVES FATIGUE.

CIRCLING ~ *YAO*

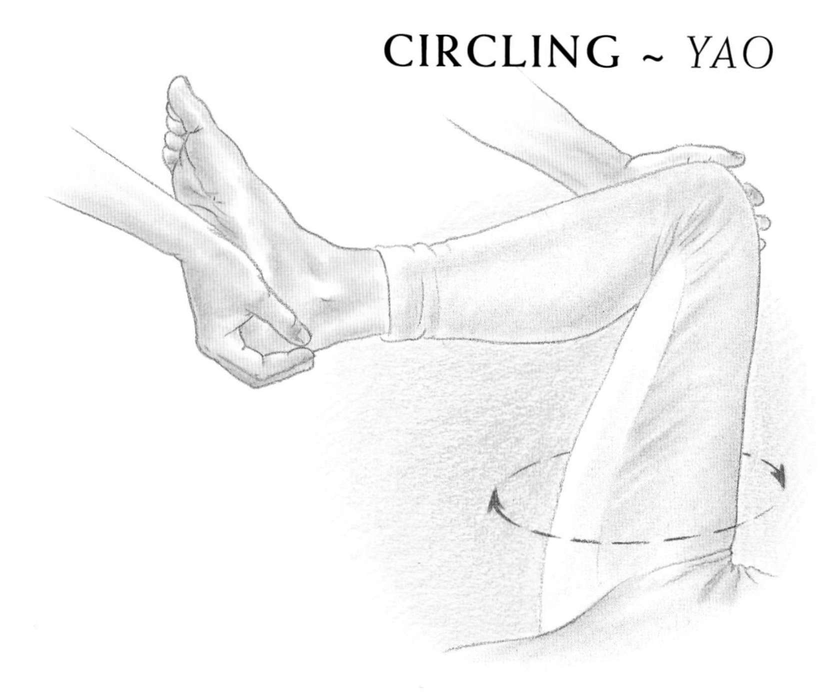

YAO applied to the leg

The Chinese circling manipulation YAO involves holding the affected limb of the patient and then circling it gently and slowly. Gradually increase the size of the circle, but not excessively or beyond the natural range of movement. YAO is usually used with DOU (see facing page).

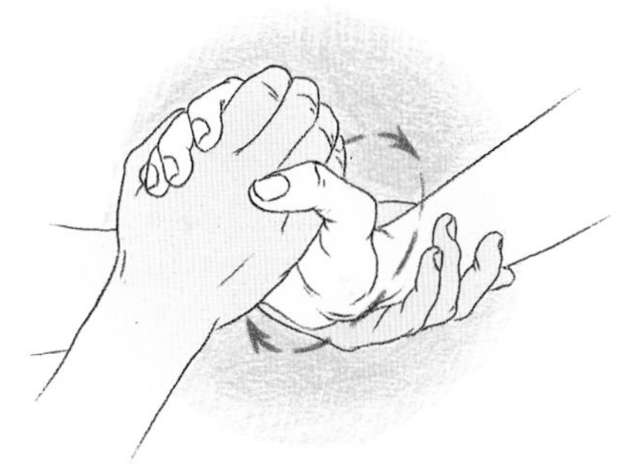

YAO applied to the wrist

USE YAO TO TREAT JOINT PROBLEMS. YAO LOOSENS STIFF JOINTS AND IMPROVES THEIR MOBILITY.

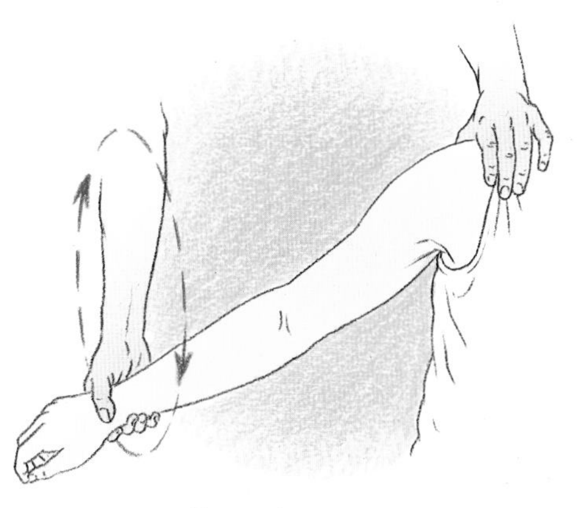

YAO applied to the arm

CHAPTER THREE

OPENING THE CHANNELS

According to traditional Chinese medicine, the channels (see pp. 8-13) form a network that carries qi-blood, and links all the vital organs and all parts of the body. When disease occurs the channels are affected, upsetting the flow of qi and blood. This disturbance is referred to as channel blockage, qi-blood stagnation, or out-of-balance yin and yang. The channels lose their normal functions, and show various symptoms of disturbance, such as pain.

Opening blocked channels lies at the heart of pain-relief massage. This chapter shows you how to do this, enabling you to remove qi-blood stagnation and to restore the balance of yin and yang. As soon as the work is done, the pain will disappear.

The method for opening the channels described in this chapter is organic. It co-ordinates and integrates the proper working of the 12 regular channels, two extra channels, and over 100 key acupoints. You can open the channels in just one region of the body or in several regions together, depending on the individual case (see chapter Four, Relieving Pain). Refer to the appendix (see pp. 122-39) to check the location of any acupoints and channels you are unsure about.

Opening the Channels in the head

Ask your partner to sit comfortably in a chair, and position yourself so that you can exert your force effectively. Remember that the acupoints on the 12 Regular Channels exist in symmetrical pairs, on each side of the body. The routine for opening the Channels in the head works on both sides of the body, using the acupoints in their pairs.

Step 1

- Squeeze and knead both UB2 (*Zanzhu*) acupoints on the inner end of each eyebrow. Massage the points with your thumb and middle finger, and repeat 20 times.
- Press the extra point *Yintang* 20 to 30 times with your thumb. Then press the acupoints Du23 (*Shangxing*), Du20 (*Baihui*), Du16 (*Fengfu*), and Du14 (*Dazhui*) 20 to 30 times each, in succession.

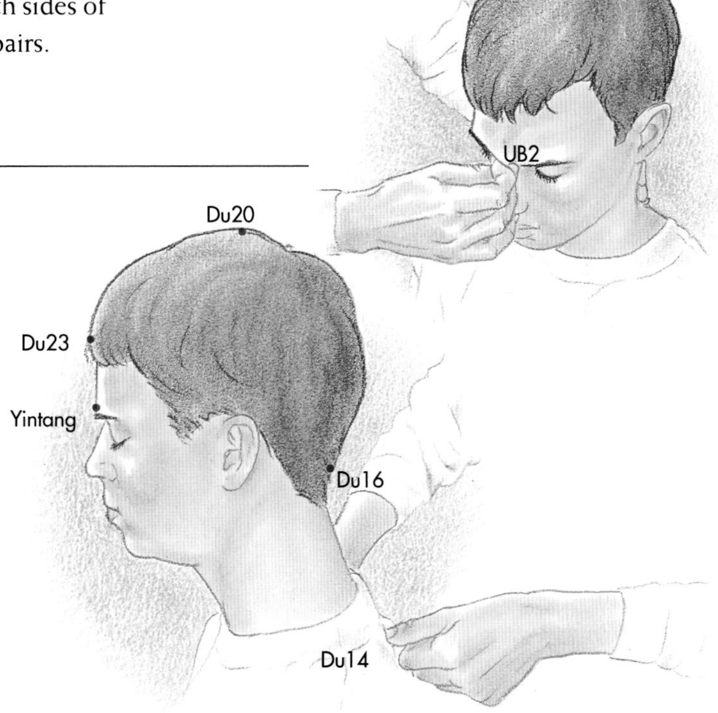

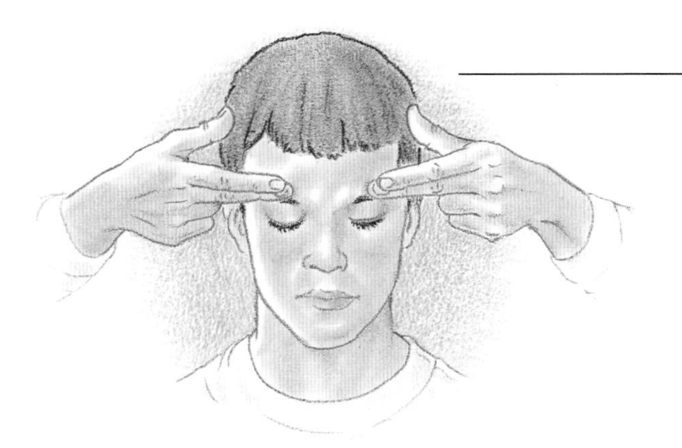

Step 2

Wipe your partner's eyebrows from the inner to the outer ends with your middle fingers. Apply smooth, even strokes, and repeat 10 times.

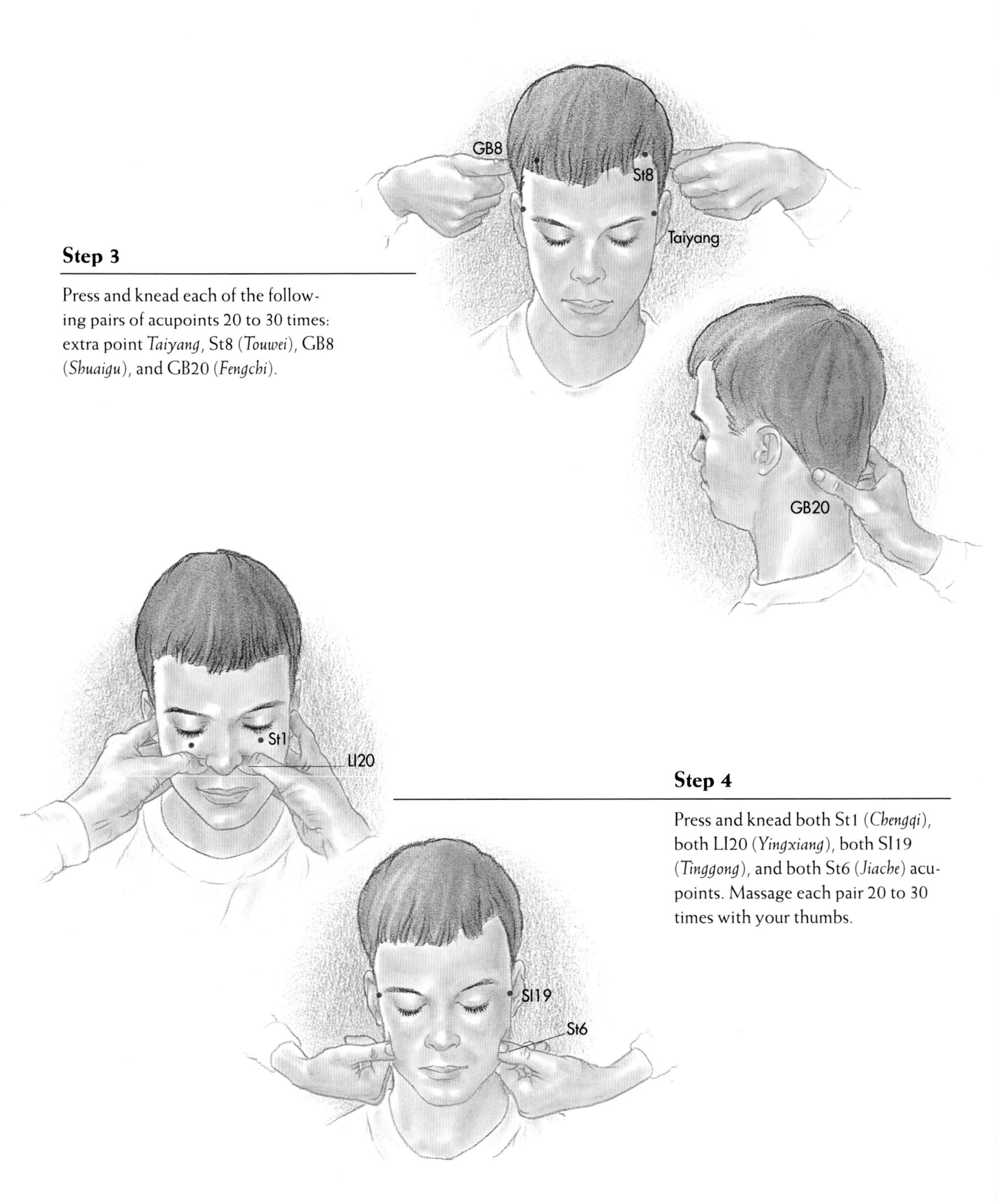

Step 3

Press and knead each of the following pairs of acupoints 20 to 30 times: extra point *Taiyang*, St8 (*Touwei*), GB8 (*Shuaigu*), and GB20 (*Fengchi*).

Step 4

Press and knead both St1 (*Chengqi*), both LI20 (*Yingxiang*), both SI19 (*Tinggong*), and both St6 (*Jiache*) acupoints. Massage each pair 20 to 30 times with your thumbs.

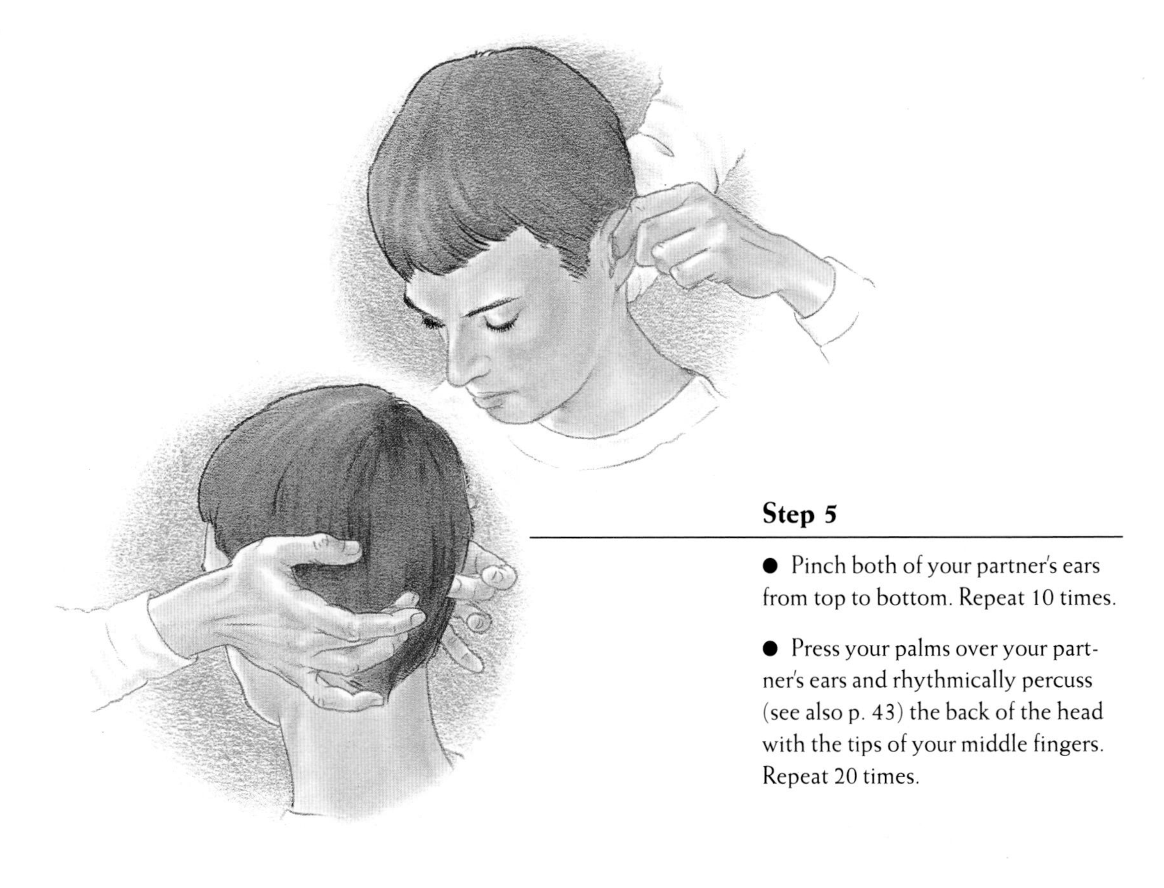

Step 5

- Pinch both of your partner's ears from top to bottom. Repeat 10 times.

- Press your palms over your partner's ears and rhythmically percuss (see also p. 43) the back of the head with the tips of your middle fingers. Repeat 20 times.

Step 6

Using the tips of your fingers, comb your partner's scalp. Start at the forehead hairline and comb to the back of the head. Repeat 20 times.

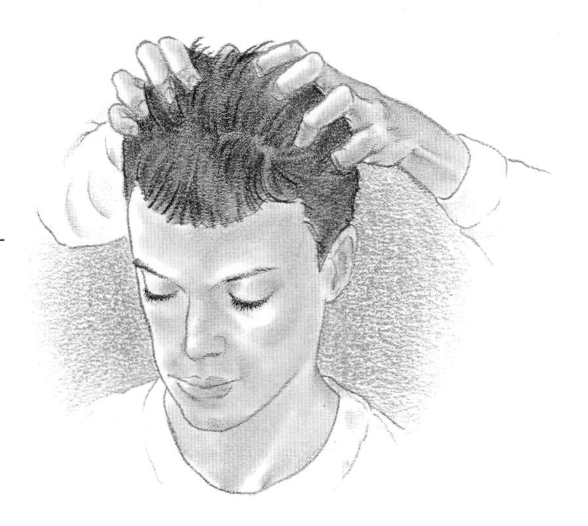

Opening the Channels in the abdomen

Your partner should lie face up, either on the floor or on a massage table for this sequence. Stand or kneel wherever is most comfortable for you to reach the required acupoints easily and apply appropriate pressure.

Step 1

Press Ren17 (*Tanzhong*) with the middle finger of your left hand. Keep pressing Ren17 while you work on acupoints Ren12 (*Zhongwan*), Ren11 (*Jianli*), Ren9 (*Shuifen*), Ren6 (*Qihai*), and Ren4 (*Guanyuan*) in succession. Use the middle finger of your right hand to press and knead each point 20 to 30 times.

Step 2

Using your palm, rub 10 clockwise circles around your partner's navel, increasing the size of the circle each time. Then rub 10 anticlockwise circles around the navel. This time, start with a large circle and reduce its size a little each time.

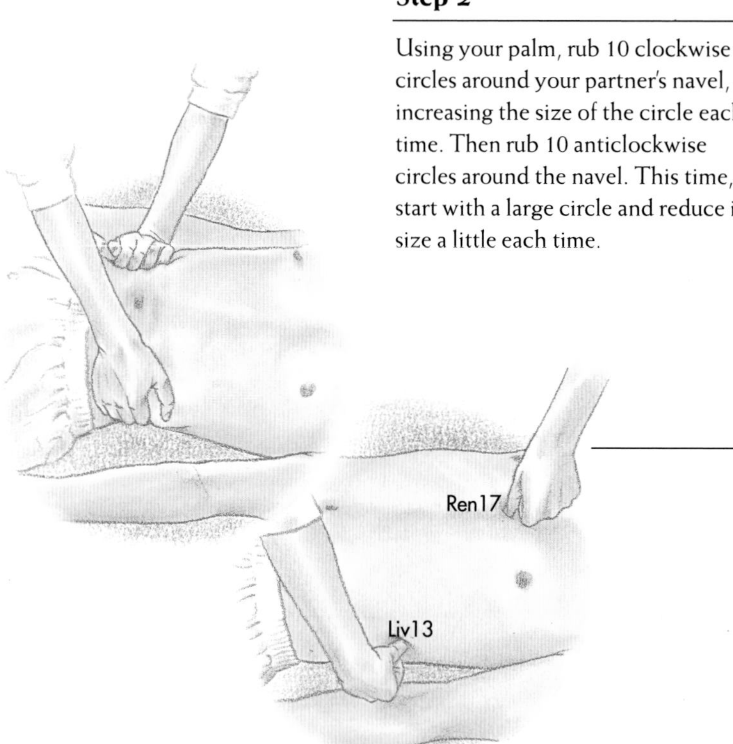

Step 3

- Hold both GB26 (*Daimai*) acupoints, then lift and fold them over the abdomen. Repeat three times.
- Press acupoint Ren17 (*Tanzhong*) on the midline of your partner's body with your thumb. At the same time, press and knead Liv13 (*Zhangmen*) on one side of the body, 20 to 30 times. Then repeat on the other side.

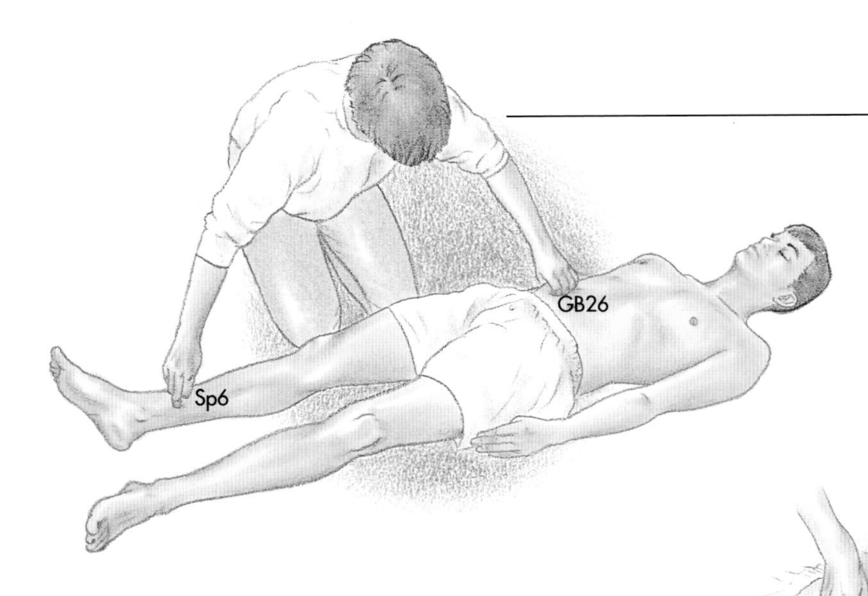

Step 4

Position yourself on your partner's right side and hold acupoint GB26 (*Daimai*) with your left hand. At the same time, press acupoint Sp6 (*Sanyinjiao*) on your partner's right leg with your right hand 20 to 30 times. Repeat the process on your partner's left side.

Step 5

● Press Ren17 (*Tanzhong*) with the thumb of your left hand. At the same time, press both St21 (*Liangmen*) acupoints and then both K18 (*Shiguan*) acupoints with your other hand. Press each pair 20 to 30 times.

● Push down the sides of your partner's body with your palms. Repeat three times.

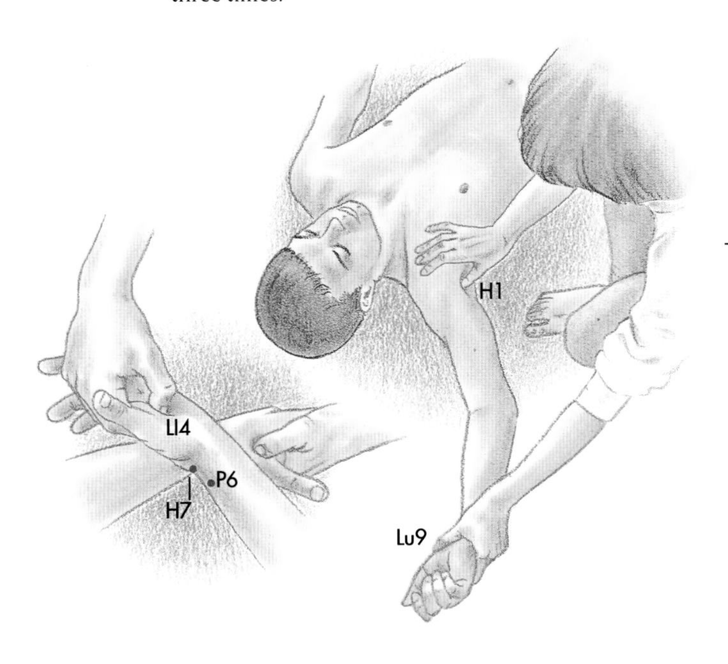

Step 6

● Raise your partner's right arm, and press acupoint Lu9 (*Taiyuan*) with your thumb. At the same time, squeeze H1 (*Jiquan*) 10 times. Then repeat the massage on the left arm.

● Press acupoints LI4 (*Hegu*), P6 (*Neiguan*), and H7 (*Shenmen*) 20 to 30 times each, in their pairs on both hands. Cross your partner's hands over for easier access to the points.

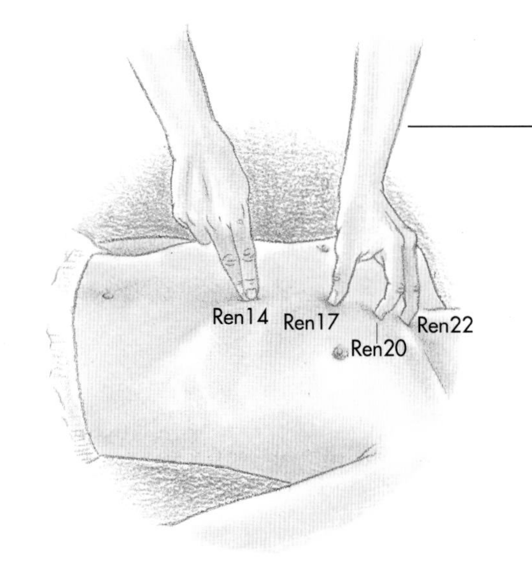

Step 7

Use the fingers of one hand to apply simultaneous pressure to acupoints Ren22 (*Tiantu*), Ren20 (*Huagai*), and Ren17 (*Tanzhong*). Keep your fingers still, and apply constant pressure. At the same time, press Ren14 (*Juque*) 20 to 30 times with the middle finger of your other hand.

Step 8

- With the thumb of one hand, press Ren14 (*Juque*). At the same time, use the fingers of your other hand to press Ren13 (*Shangwan*), Ren12 (*Zhongwan*), and Ren10 (*Xiawan*). Press all four acupoints together, 20 to 30 times.

- Use the middle finger of one hand to press Ren12 (*Zhongwan*). At the same time, use the middle finger of your other hand to knead acupoints Ren6 (*Qihai*), Ren4 (*Guanyuan*), and Ren3 (*Zhongji*) in succession. Knead each acupoint 20 to 30 times.

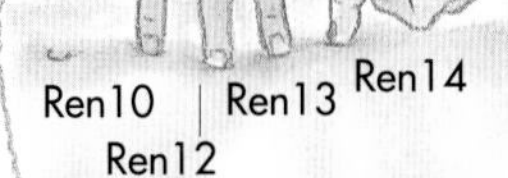

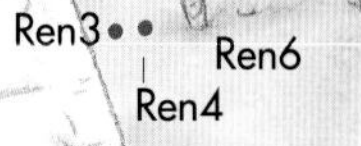

St25
St21

Step 9

Using the thumb and index finger of each hand, knead both St21 (*Liangmen*) and both St25 (*Tianshu*) acupoints simultaneously. Repeat 20 to 30 times.

Step 10

- Press Ren15 (*Jiuwei*) with your thumb. At the same time, use the thumb and middle finger of your other hand to squeeze acupoints GB34 (*Yanglingquan*) and Sp9 (*Yinlingquan*) together on one leg. Squeeze the points 20 to 30 times, and then repeat the sequence on the other leg.
- Press acupoint Lu1 (*Zhongfu*) on both sides of your partner's body 20 to 30 times with your thumbs.

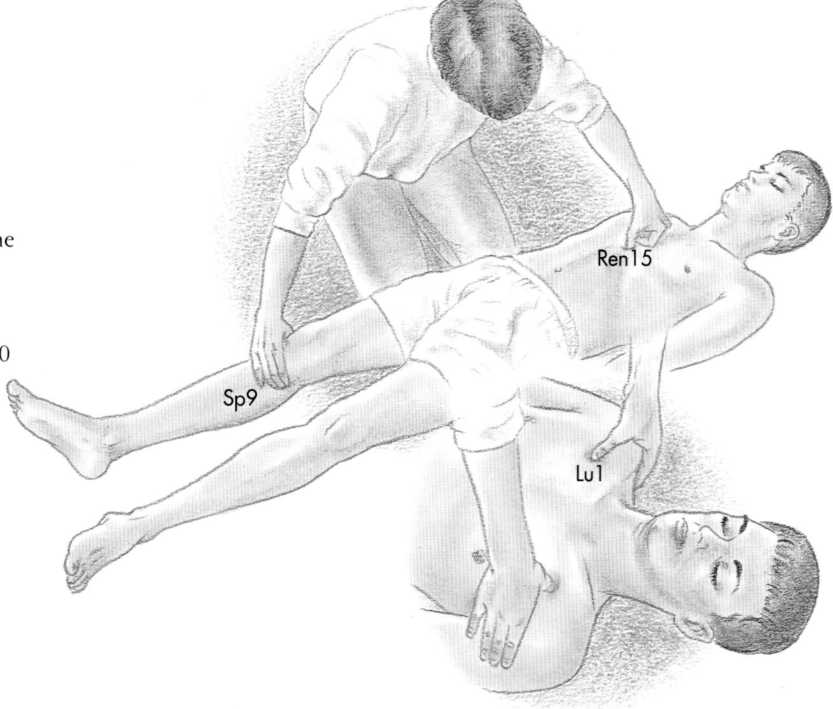

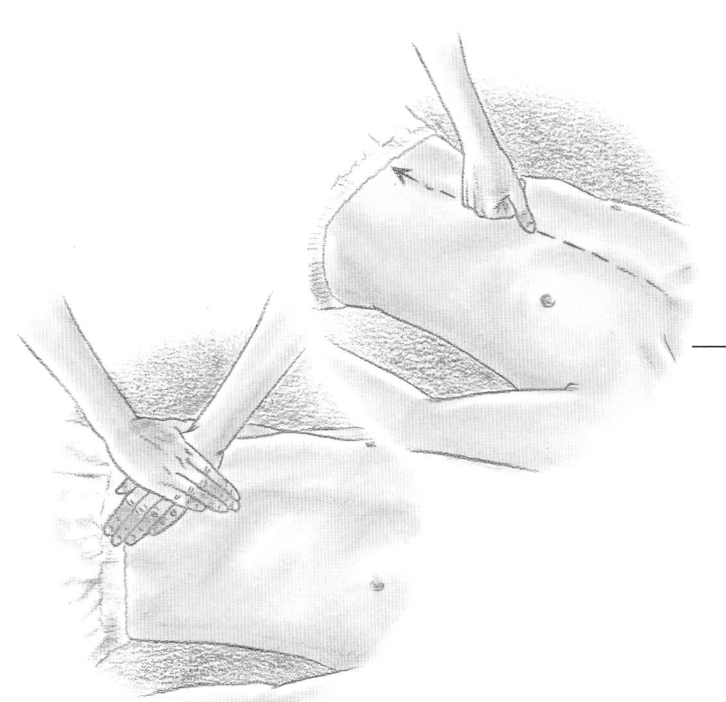

Step 11

- Using your thumb, slowly push down the midline of your partner's body along the Ren Channel. Start at Ren22 (*Tiantu*) at the top of the breastbone, and push down to Ren3 (*Zhongji*). Repeat five times.
- Place your hands, one on top of the other, on your partner's navel. Apply pressure and quiver your hands with a rapid movement (see also p. 41).

Opening the Channels in the back

Use this sequence to relieve back pain. You can also practise this back sequence together with opening the Channels in the abdomen (see pp. 50-3) to treat pain and disease of the internal organs. Similarly, practise this back sequence with the method of opening the Channels in the leg (see pp. 61-3) to relieve leg pain.

Step 1

Kneel or stand at your partner's head and rub the back with your palms using broad, smooth strokes. This step helps to relax the back muscles.

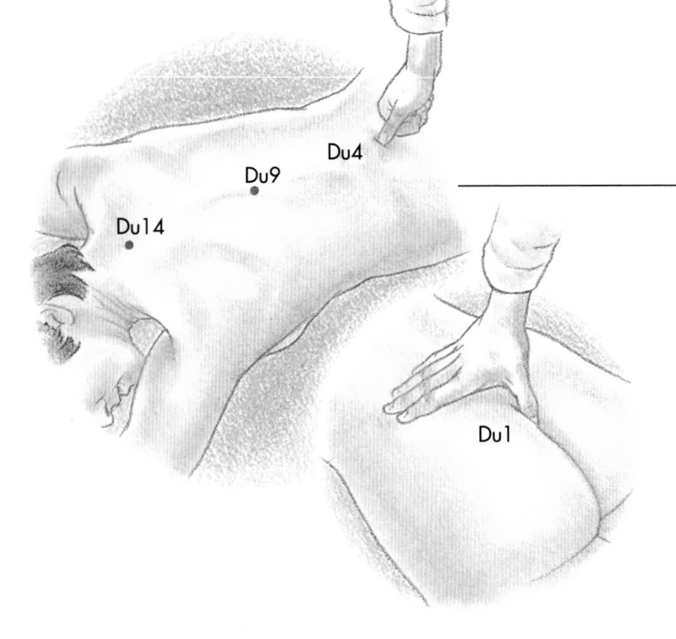

Step 2

- Press acupoints Du14 (*Dazhui*), Du9 (*Zhiyang*), and Du4 (*Mingmen*) in turn with your thumb. Press the points 20 to 30 times each.

- Press acupoint Du1 (*Changqiang*) with your thumb for three minutes. Since this point is located midway between the coccyx and the anus, you should be particularly aware of your partner's need for privacy. If preferred, press this point through thin cotton underwear.

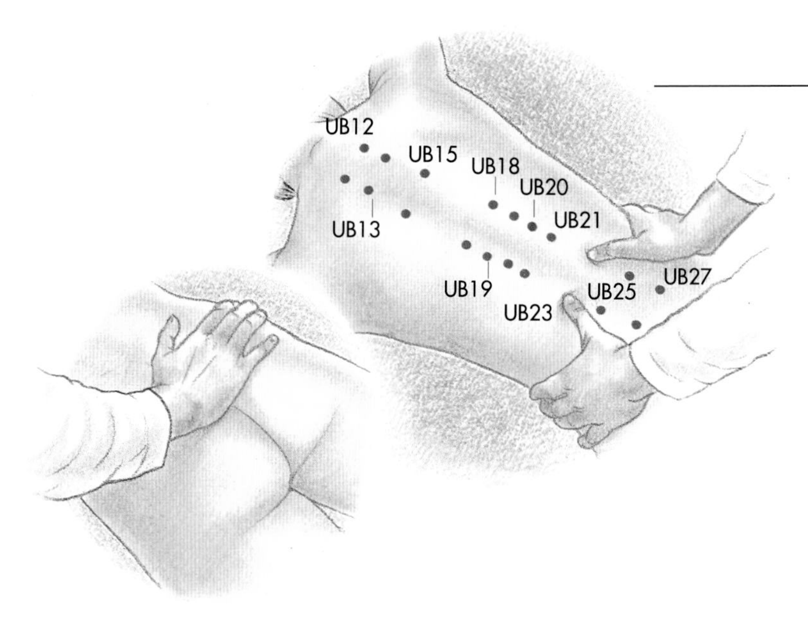

Step 3

- Press the following pairs of acupoints on both Urinary Bladder Channels: UB12 (*Fengmen*), UB13 (*Feishu*), UB15 (*Xinshu*), UB18 (*Ganshu*), UB19 (*Danshu*), UB20 (*Pishu*), UB21 (*Weishu*), UB23 (*Shenshu*), UB25 (*Dachangshu*), and UB27 (*Xiaochangshu*). Press each pair 20 to 30 times with your thumbs.
- Press the group of eight acupoints on the Urinary Bladder Channel that are collectively known as UB31-34 (*Baliao*). Press the points with the heel of your hand 20 to 30 times. Then repeat from the other side of your partner's body.

Step 4

Work down both of your partner's legs pressing the following successive pairs of acupoints: GB30 (*Huantiao*), UB37 (*Yinmen*), UB40 (*Weizhong*), UB57 (*Chengshan*), UB60 (*Kunlun*), and K1 (*Yongquan*). Press each pair 20 to 30 times with your thumbs.

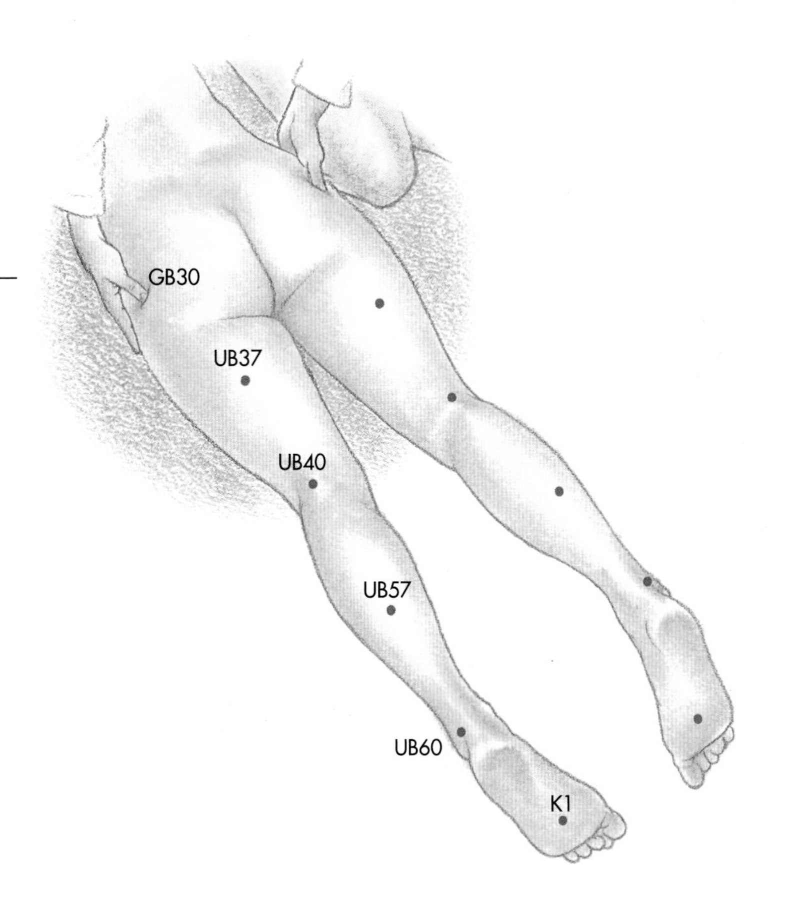

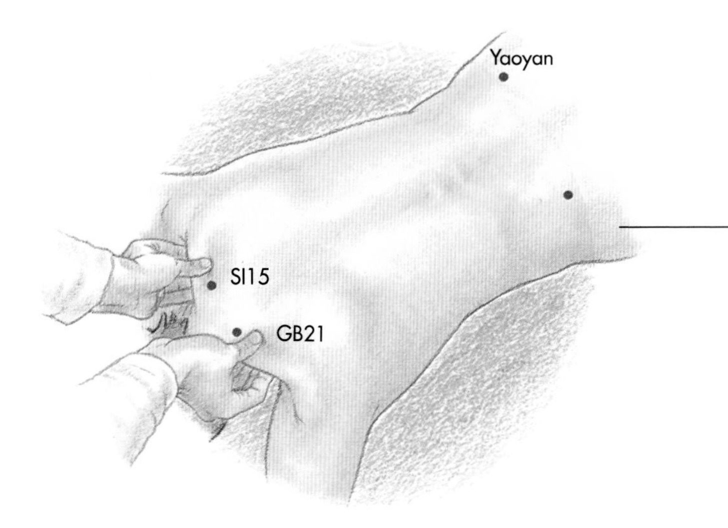

Step 5

- Squeeze both GB21 (*Jianjing*) acupoints with your thumbs and fingers 20 to 30 times.

- Press both SI15 (*Jianzhongshu*) acupoints 20 to 30 times, with your thumbs.

- Rub both extra *Yaoyan* acupoints with your palms for one to two minutes.

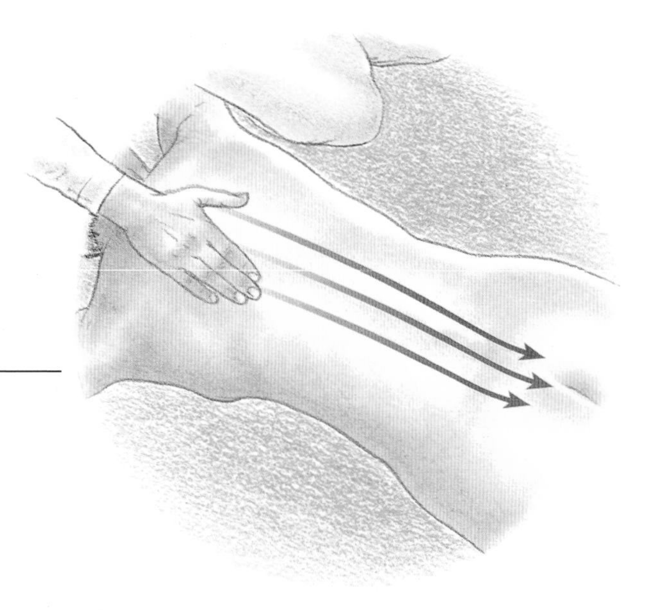

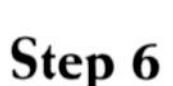

Step 6

- Use your palm to press and push down the Du Channel from Du14 (*Dazhui*) to the coccyx. Apply firm pressure, and repeat five times.

- Then use your palm to press and push down the Urinary Bladder Channel on one side of the spine. Start at UB12 (*Fengmen*) and end at UB31-34 (*Baliao*). Repeat five times. Then repeat on the Urinary Bladder Channel on the other side of the spine.

Opening the Channels in the arm

Your partner should sit in a comfortable chair while you open the Channels in the arm. This sequence works on the three Yang Channels and the three Yin Channels of the Hand. Perform the whole sequence on the affected arm. Then, if necessary, repeat the sequence on the other arm.

Step 1

- Squeeze both the GB21 (*Jianjing*) acupoints on your partner's shoulders. Squeeze the points firmly 30 times.
- Work down the Large Intestine Channel of your partner's affected arm pressing the following acupoints one by one: LI15 (*Jianyu*), LI14 (*Binao*), LI11 (*Quchi*), LI10 (*Shousanli*), LI5 (*Yangxi*), LI4 (*Hegu*), and LI1 (*Shangyang*). Press each point 20 to 30 times with your thumb.

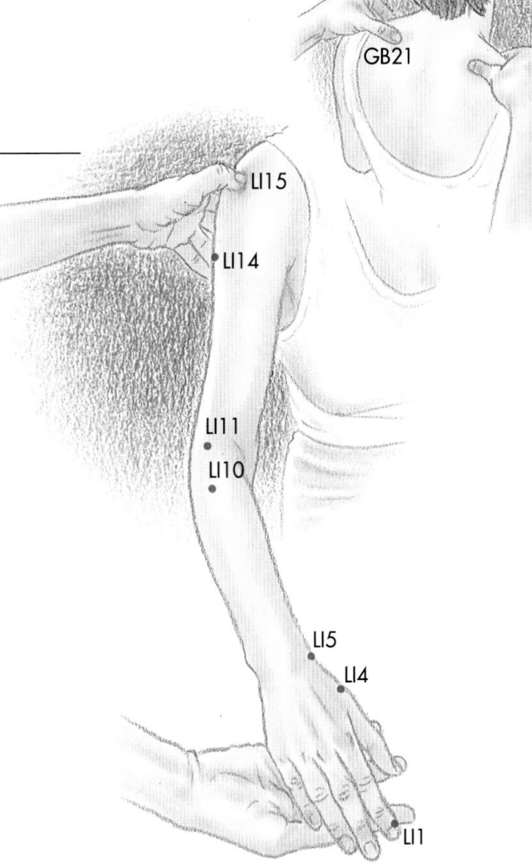

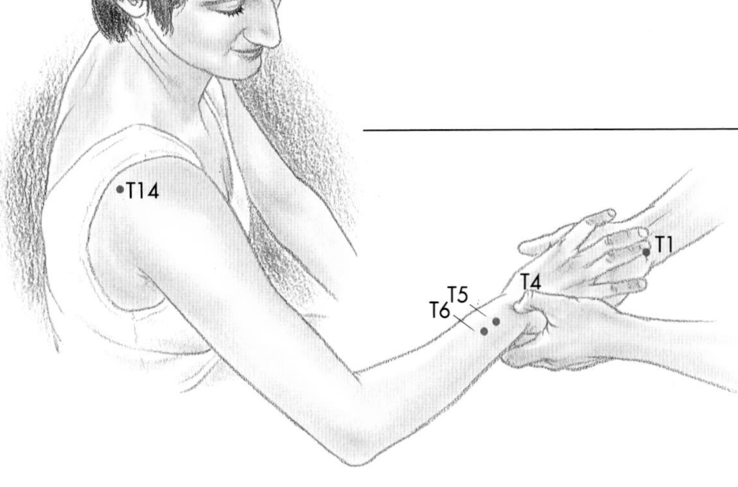

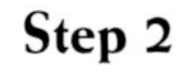

Step 2

Using your thumb, press the following acupoints on the Triple Warmer Channel: T14 (*Jianliao*), T6 (*Zhigou*), T5 (*Waiguan*), T4 (*Yangchi*), and T1 (*Guanchong*). Press each point 20 to 30 times in turn.

Step 3

In sequence, press acupoints SI11 (*Tianzong*), SI9 (*Jianzhen*), SI8 (*Xiaohai*), SI3 (*Houxi*), and SI1 (*Shaoze*) on the Small Intestine Channel. Press each point 20 to 30 times with your thumb.

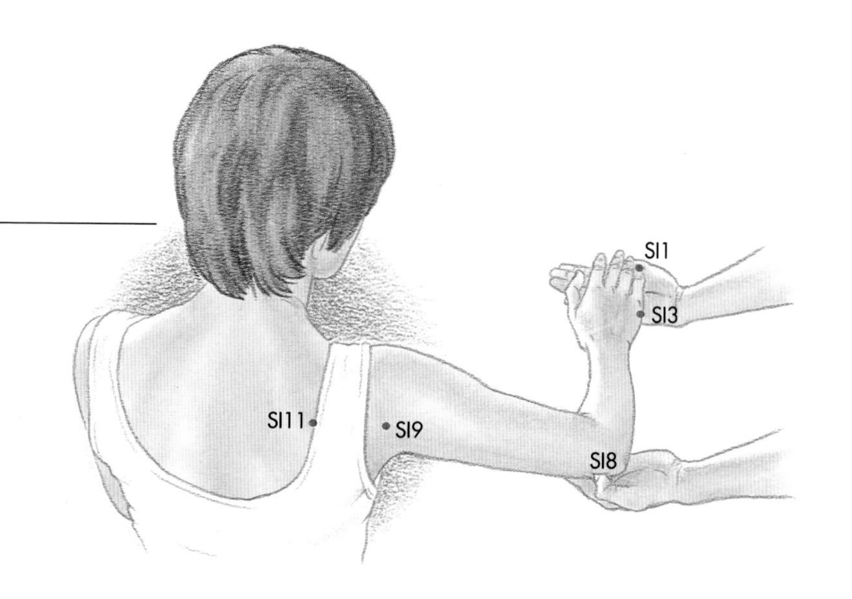

Step 4

Open the Lung Channel by pressing acupoints Lu5 (*Chize*), Lu7 (*Lieque*), Lu9 (*Taiyuan*), Lu10 (*Yuji*), and Lu11 (*Shaoshang*) with your thumb. Press the points one by one, 20 to 30 times each.

Step 5

With your thumb, press P3 (*Quze*), P6 (*Neiguan*), P8 (*Laogong*), and P9 (*Zhongchong*) acupoints on the Pericardium Channel. Press the points 20 to 30 times each, in succession.

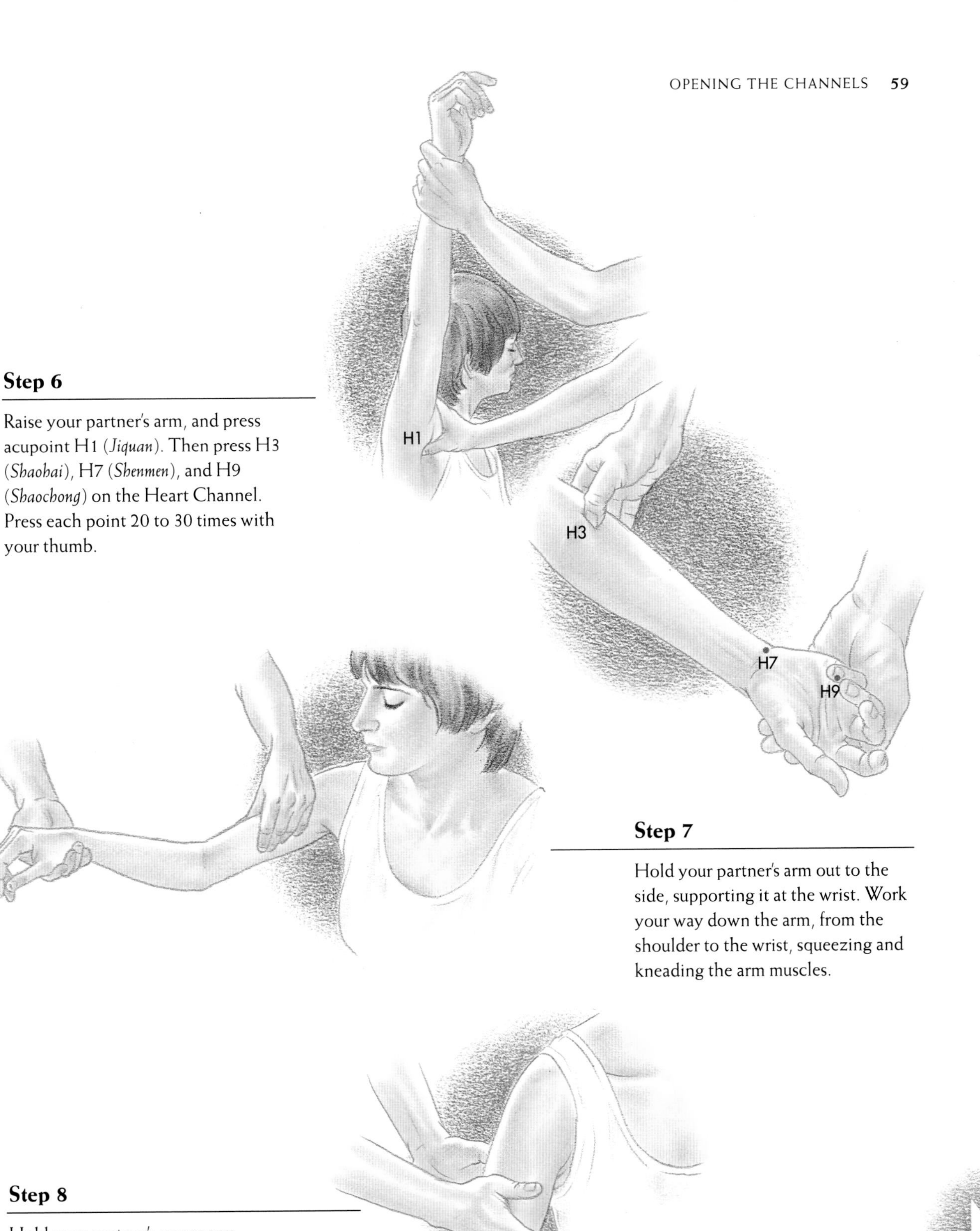

Step 6

Raise your partner's arm, and press acupoint H1 (*Jiquan*). Then press H3 (*Shaohai*), H7 (*Shenmen*), and H9 (*Shaochong*) on the Heart Channel. Press each point 20 to 30 times with your thumb.

Step 7

Hold your partner's arm out to the side, supporting it at the wrist. Work your way down the arm, from the shoulder to the wrist, squeezing and kneading the arm muscles.

Step 8

Hold your partner's upper arm between your palms, and twist it by moving your palms back and forth in opposite directions (see also p. 43).

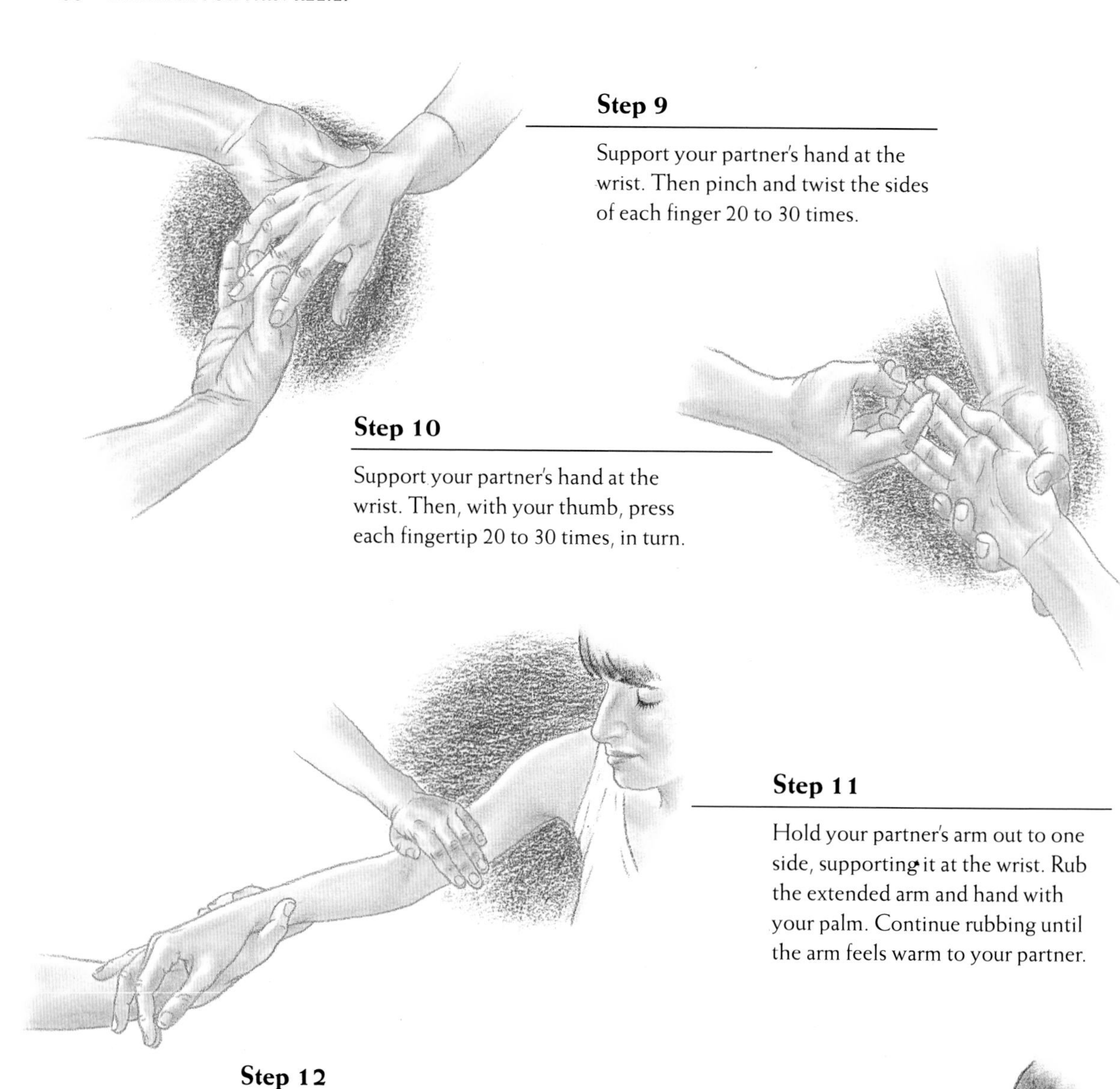

Step 9

Support your partner's hand at the wrist. Then pinch and twist the sides of each finger 20 to 30 times.

Step 10

Support your partner's hand at the wrist. Then, with your thumb, press each fingertip 20 to 30 times, in turn.

Step 11

Hold your partner's arm out to one side, supporting it at the wrist. Rub the extended arm and hand with your palm. Continue rubbing until the arm feels warm to your partner.

Step 12

Place one hand on your partner's shoulder and hold the wrist firmly with your other hand. Shake the arm up and down in a wave-like motion ten times (see also p. 44).

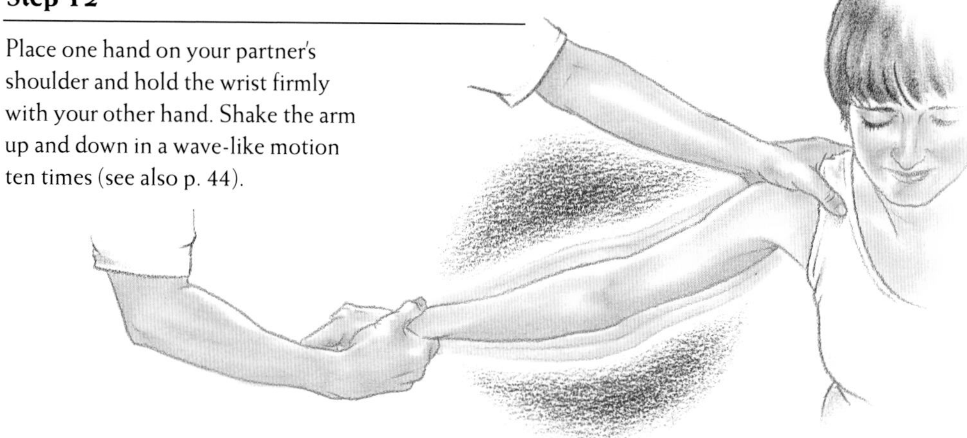

Opening the Channels in the leg

Your partner should be lying down for this sequence, which works on the three Yang Channels and three Yin Channels of the Leg. Practise the whole sequence on the affected leg. Then, if necessary, repeat the sequence on the other leg.

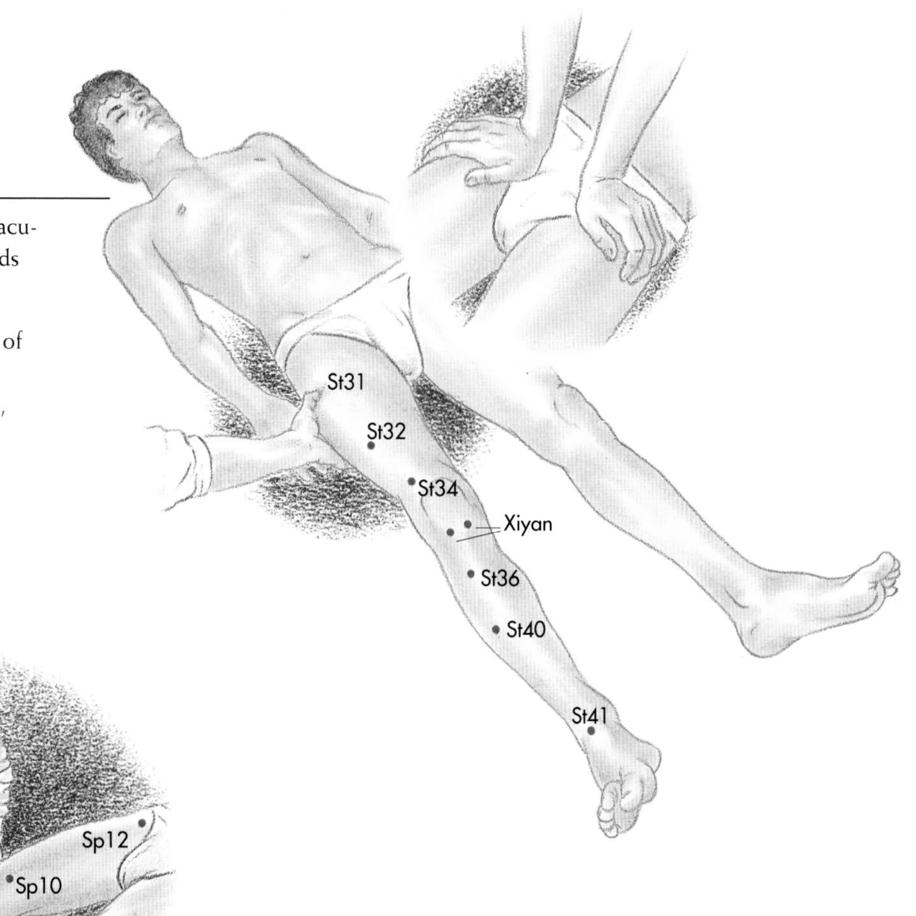

Step 1

- Press both the St30 (*Qichong*) acupoints with the heels of your hands for two minutes.
- Using your thumb, press each of the following acupoints 20 to 30 times in succession: St31 (*Biguan*), St32 (*Futu*), St34 (*Liangqiu*), extra points *Xiyan*, St36 (*Zusanli*), St40 (*Fenglong*), and St41 (*Jiexi*).

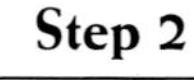

Step 2

One by one, press the following acupoints on the Spleen Channel: Sp12 (*Chongmen*), Sp10 (*Xuehai*), Sp9 (*Yinlingquan*), Sp6 (*Sanyinjiao*), and Sp4 (*Gongsun*). Press each point 20 to 30 times with your thumb.

Step 3

Press acupoints GB30 (*Huantiao*), GB31 (*Fengshi*), GB34 (*Yanglingquan*), GB39 (*Xuanzhong*), and GB40 (*Qiuxu*) in succession on the Gall Bladder Channel. Use your thumbs, and press each point 20 to 30 times.

Step 4

Work down the Urinary Bladder Channel with your thumb, pressing acupoints UB36 (*Chengfu*), UB37 (*Yinmen*), UB40 (*Weizhong*), UB57 (*Chengshan*), and UB60 (*Kunlun*). Press the points, one by one, 20 to 30 times each.

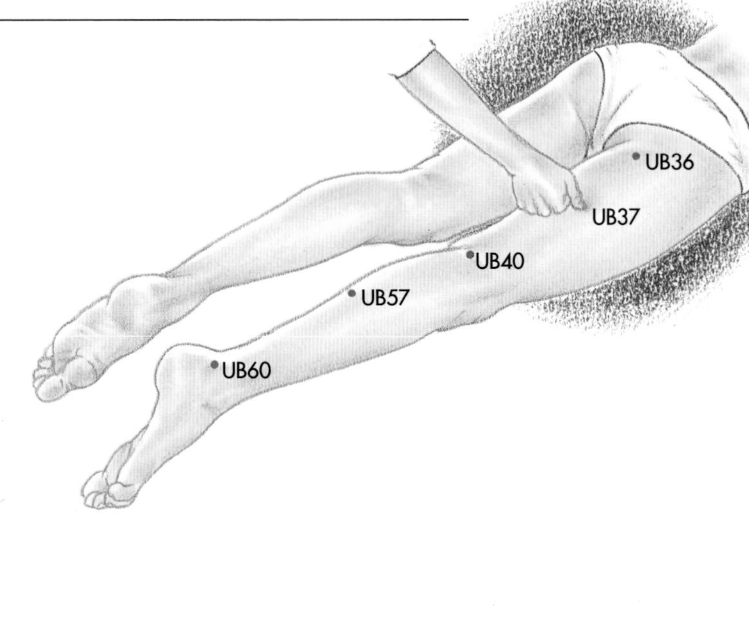

Step 5

Use your thumb to press acupoints K3 (*Taixi*), K6 (*Zhaohai*), and K1 (*Yongquan*) in succession on the Kidney Channel. Press each point 20 to 30 times.

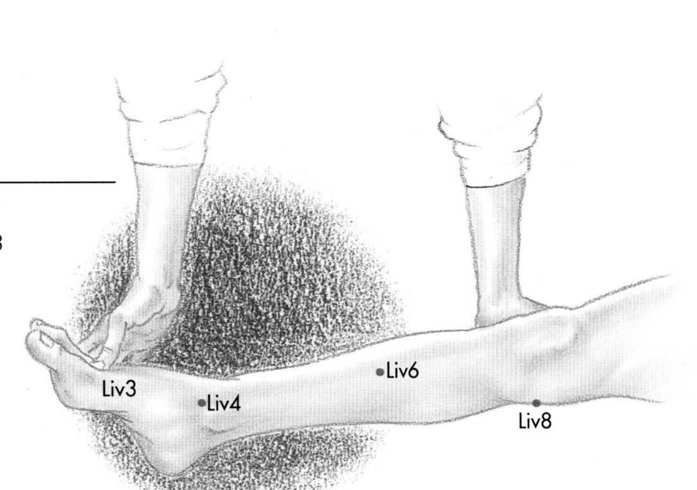

Step 6

Press acupoints Liv8 (*Ququan*), Liv6 (*Zhongdu*), Liv4 (*Zhongfeng*), and Liv3 (*Taichong*), one by one, on the Liver Channel. Press each point 20 to 30 times with your thumb.

Step 7

Work your way down your partner's leg, squeezing the leg muscles with both hands.

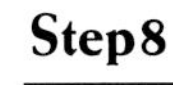

Step8

Support your partner's foot, and with your other hand pinch and knead the sides of each toe in turn. Repeat 20 to 30 times for each toe.

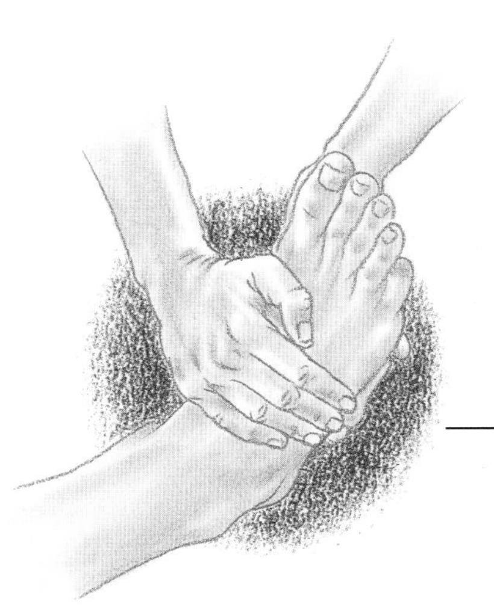

Step 9

Rub up and down over the top of the foot, with your palm. Repeat 20 times.

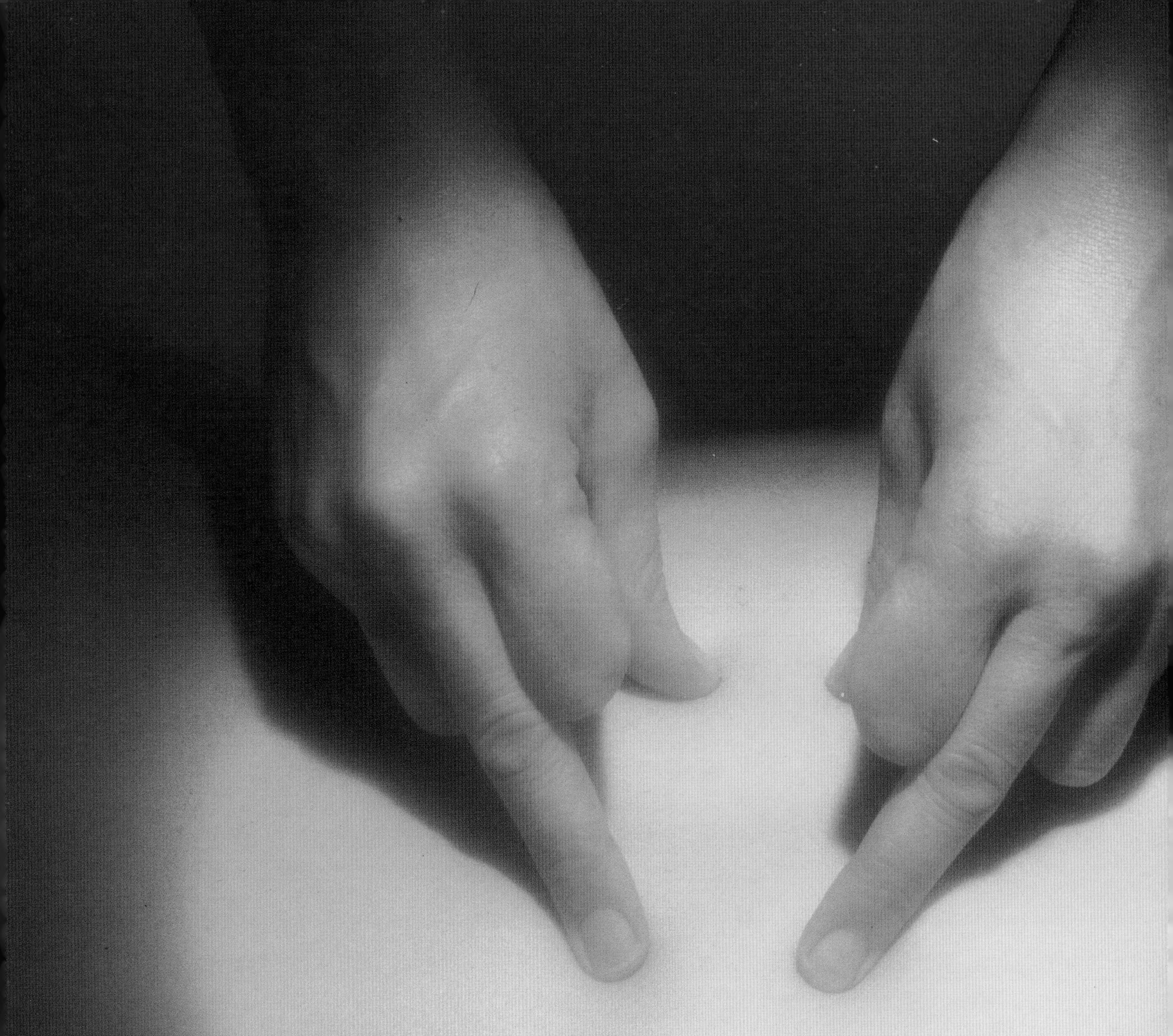

part two

THE PRACTICE

CHAPTER FOUR

RELIEVING PAIN

In this chapter you practise the skills that you learned earlier in the book in order to treat a wide range of painful diseases and conditions. Refer to chapter two for details of any of the massage strokes, and turn to the appendix to verify the location of any point or channel.

Since opening the channels is the basis of pain-relief massage, many of the treatments include one or more steps to do just this, and you should follow the appropriate sequence outlined in chapter three. However, you will often need to press some points – referred to as major acupoints – a few more times than others in a sequence. In most cases, press these major acupoints 30 to 40 times each, instead of 20 to 30 times.

If pain exists on one side of the body, treat the channels and points on the same side (or on both sides in some cases). If pain occurs on both sides, or on the central part of the body, work on the symmetrical pairs of channels and points on both sides of the body.

You need not adhere rigidly to these treatments – adapt them to your partner's specific needs. You can also use them for reference when treating other painful conditions which are not mentioned in this book.

HEADACHE

Headaches have a multitude of causes. A common cause is stress, which creates tension in the shoulders, neck, and head. Others include high blood pressure, insomnia, sinus congestion, the common cold, anxiety, fatigue, anaemia, eye-strain, alcohol, and migraine.

According to Chinese medicine, a headache is caused by deficient Qi and blood, or an invasion of excess Yang in the Liver. The massage routines below are classified according to where the pain is felt, but each treatment will effectively relieve any painful headache, whatever the cause. In every case, start the treatment by following the three steps for general headaches, and then apply the specific steps according to where your partner feels pain, and the cause of the headache.

General headache ~ Step 1

To relieve the pain of any headache, start by opening the Channels in the head region (see pp. 47-9). This helps to restore the Qi-blood flow to its normal situation, and to rebalance Yin and Yang.

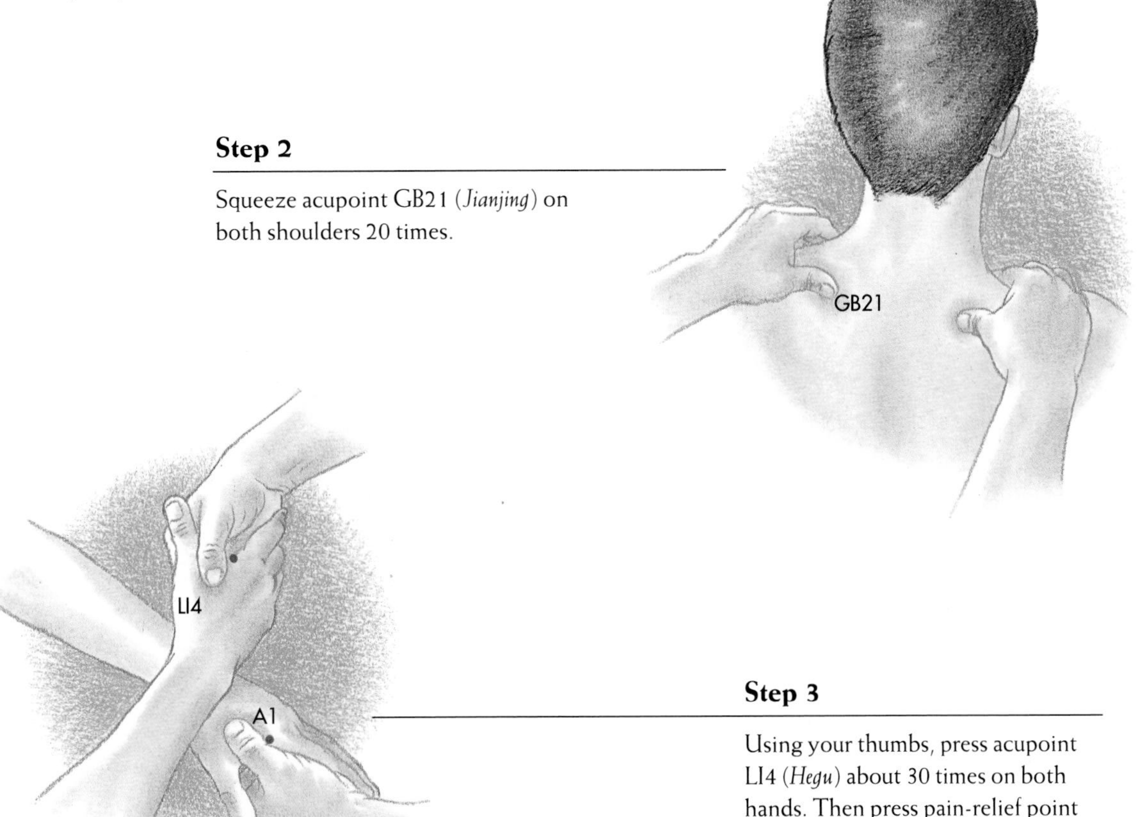

Step 2

Squeeze acupoint GB21 (*Jianjing*) on both shoulders 20 times.

Step 3

Using your thumbs, press acupoint LI4 (*Hegu*) about 30 times on both hands. Then press pain-relief point A1 on both hands for three minutes.

For headaches in the forehead

Start by following Steps 1 to 3 for general headache (see p. 67). Apply finger and thumb pressure to acupoint GB14 (*Yangbai*) on both sides of the forehead, and repeat 30 times. Then apply thumb pressure to pain-relief point B1 on both arms for two minutes.

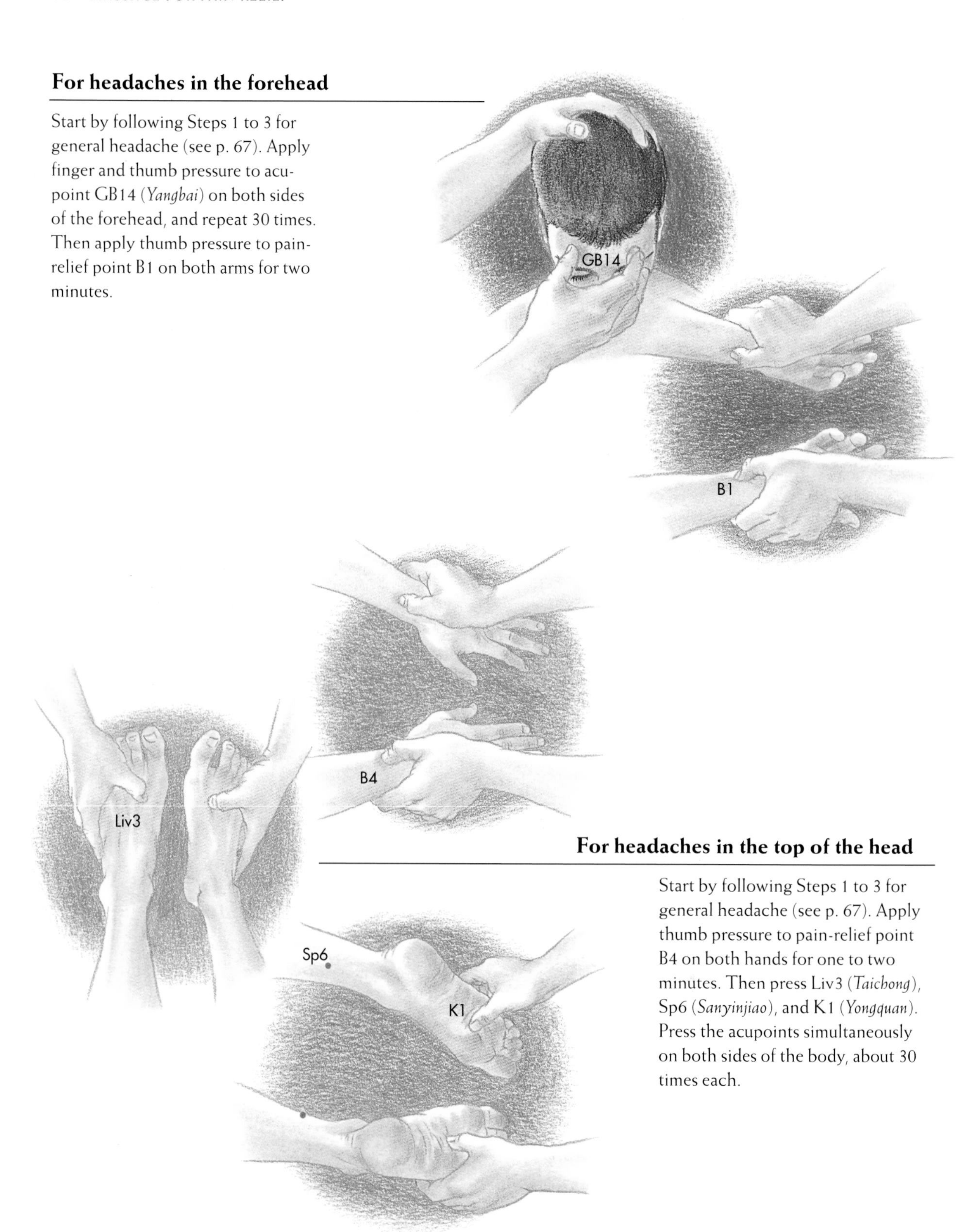

For headaches in the top of the head

Start by following Steps 1 to 3 for general headache (see p. 67). Apply thumb pressure to pain-relief point B4 on both hands for one to two minutes. Then press Liv3 (*Taichong*), Sp6 (*Sanyinjiao*), and K1 (*Yongquan*). Press the acupoints simultaneously on both sides of the body, about 30 times each.

For headaches in the back of the head

Start by performing Steps 1 to 3 for general headache (see p. 67). Then apply thumb pressure to acupoints UB10 (*Tianzhu*), SI3 (*Houxi*), P6 (*Neiguan*), T5 (*Waiguan*), and Lu7 (*Lieque*) in succession. Press the points simultaneously on both sides of the body, about 30 times each. Then press pain-relief point B6 on both wrists for one to two minutes.

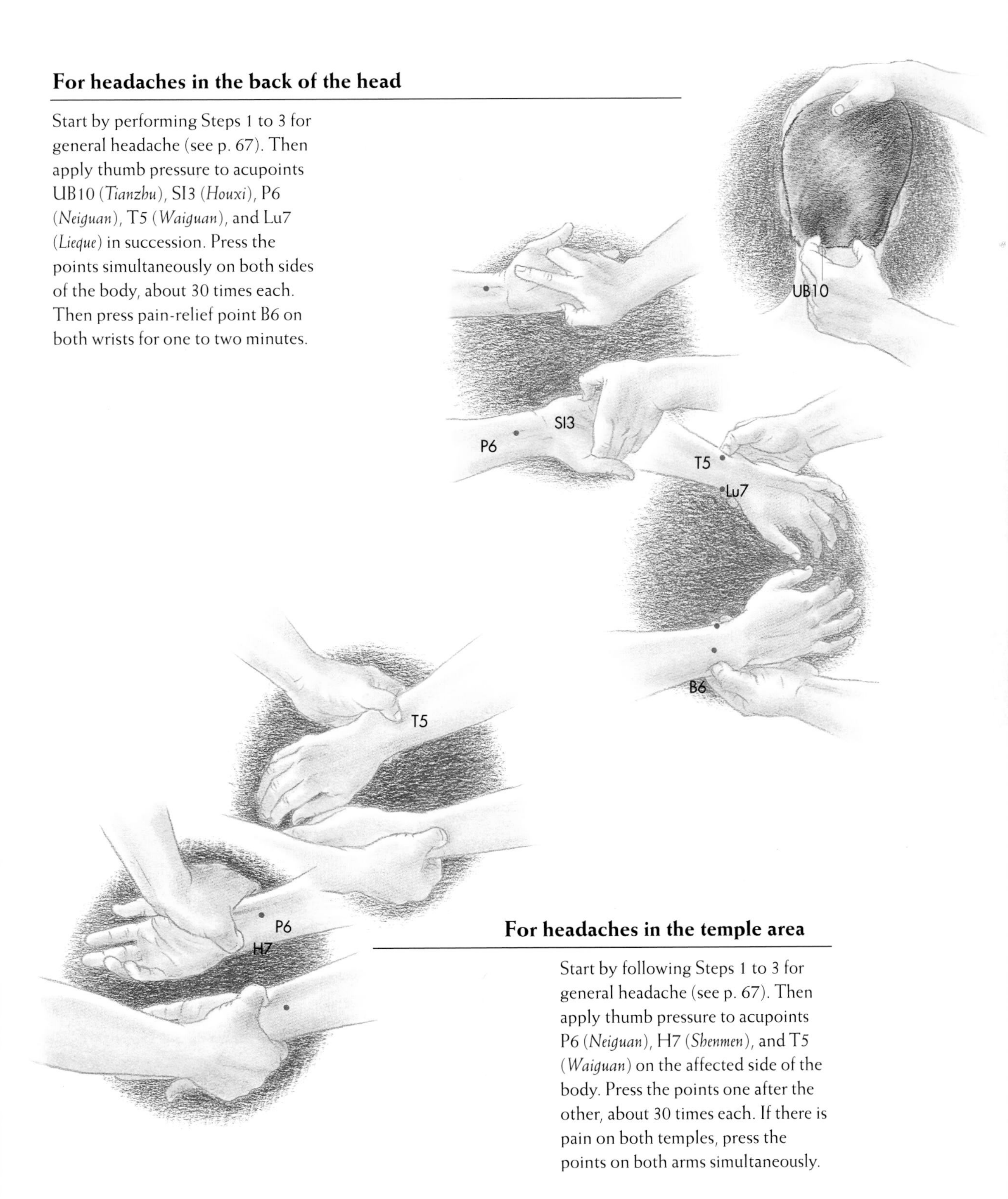

For headaches in the temple area

Start by following Steps 1 to 3 for general headache (see p. 67). Then apply thumb pressure to acupoints P6 (*Neiguan*), H7 (*Shenmen*), and T5 (*Waiguan*) on the affected side of the body. Press the points one after the other, about 30 times each. If there is pain on both temples, press the points on both arms simultaneously.

For headache caused by high blood pressure, insomnia, neurosis, or nervousness

Start by performing Steps 1 to 3 for general headache (see p. 67). Then apply thumb pressure to extra point *Anmian*, LI11 (*Quchi*), P6 (*Neiguan*), H7 (*Shenmen*), St36 (*Zusanli*), Sp6 (*Sanyinjiao*), and K1 (*Yongquan*) on both sides of the body. Press the acupoints in succession, about 30 times each. Then press pain-relief point B3 on both arms for one to two minutes.

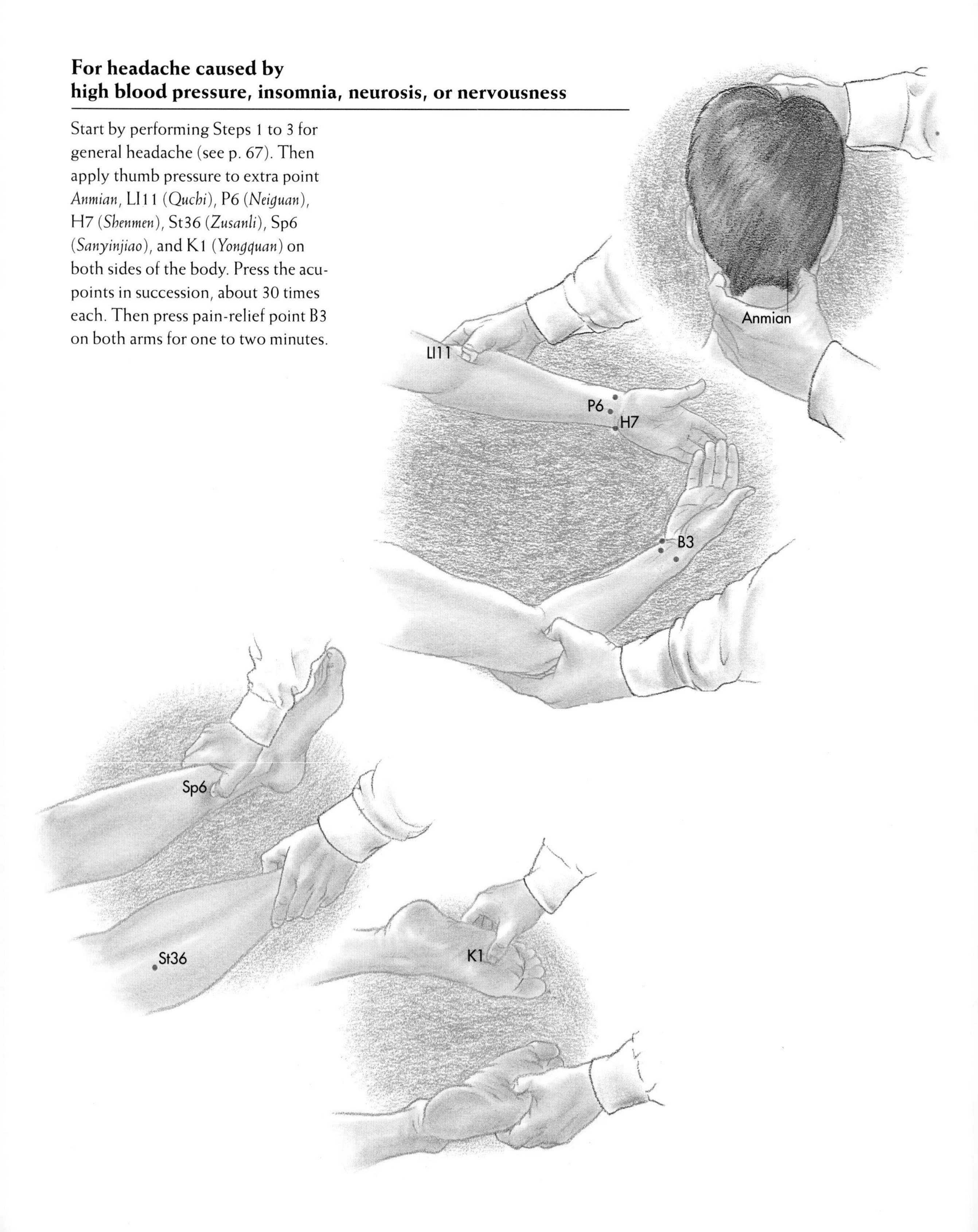

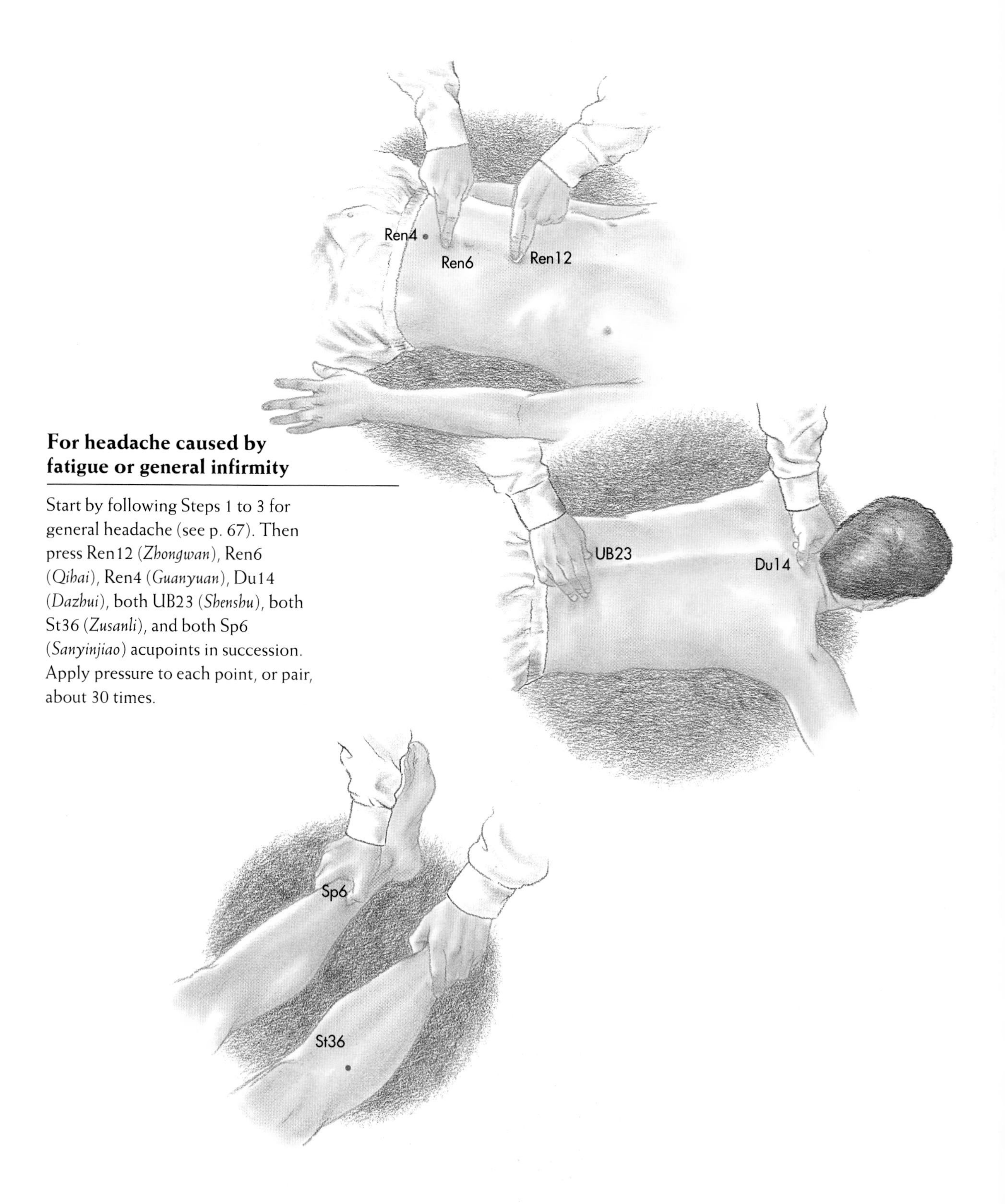

For headache caused by fatigue or general infirmity

Start by following Steps 1 to 3 for general headache (see p. 67). Then press Ren12 (*Zhongwan*), Ren6 (*Qihai*), Ren4 (*Guanyuan*), Du14 (*Dazhui*), both UB23 (*Shenshu*), both St36 (*Zusanli*), and both Sp6 (*Sanyinjiao*) acupoints in succession. Apply pressure to each point, or pair, about 30 times.

TOOTHACHE

The intensity of toothache varies from a dull ache to intense pain. The pain may also be recurring. Toothache is commonly caused by tooth decay, gum disease, or an abscess. In all cases, arrange to see your dentist as soon as possible, but in the meantime, massage can help relieve the pain. Massage the points on the same side of the body as the toothache, although you can press the pain-relief points on both sides of the body.

General toothache ~ Step 1

Your partner can be seated for this massage. Press LI4 (*Hegu*), the main acupoint for treating pains in the head region, and then pain-relief points A1 and C on the hand. Press the points firmly, one by one, for two to three minutes each.

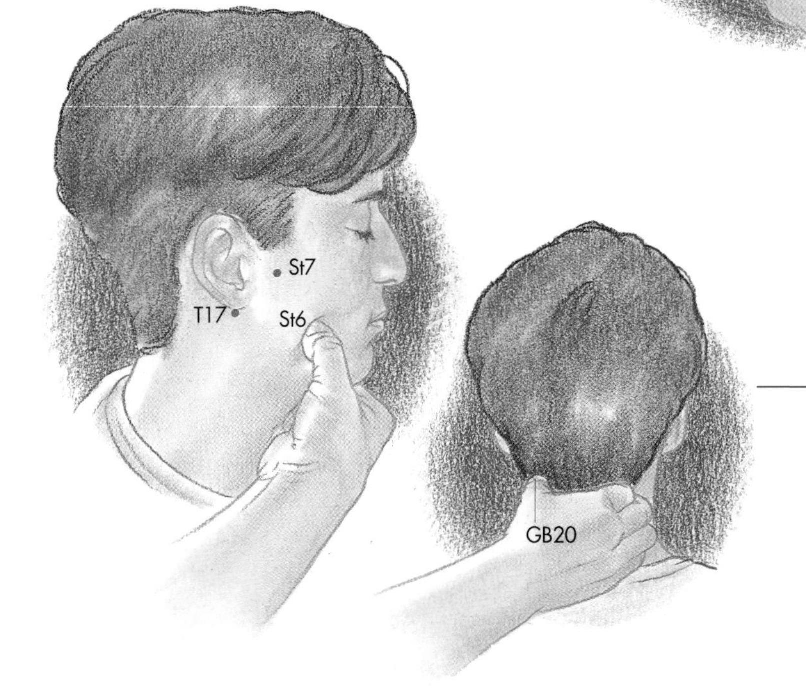

Step 2

With your thumbs, press acupoints St7 (*Xiaguan*), St6 (*Jiache*), and T17 (*Yifeng*) on the affected side of the face. Press the points one by one, 40 to 50 times each. Then press both GB20 (*Fengchi*) acupoints at the back of the head, 40 to 50 times.

Toothache of the upper jaw

Apply thumb pressure to both LI20 (*Yingxiang*) acupoints, both St2 (*Sibai*) acupoints, and Du26 (*Renzhong*), 40 to 50 times each.

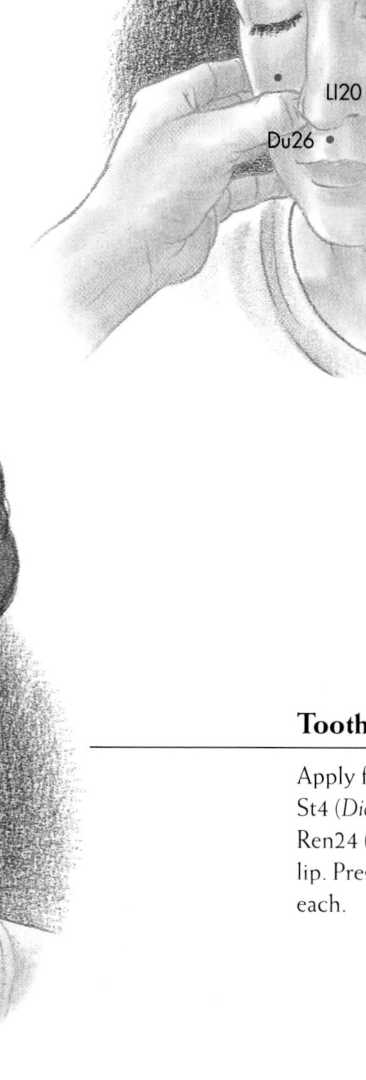

Toothache of the lower jaw

Apply firm thumb pressure to both St4 (*Dicang*) acupoints, and then to Ren24 (*Chengjiang*) under the lower lip. Press the points 40 to 50 times each.

TRIGEMINAL NEURALGIA

This is a severe and often very painful form of neuralgia that affects the trigeminal nerve and its branches on the face. It is characterized by an intensely sharp and cutting pain, and the affected area is stiff, tender to the touch, and may be red.

According to Chinese medicine, this problem is often caused by Qi-blood stagnation in the face, or an imbalance of Yin and Yang: Yin is weak and insubstantial, and there is an excess of Yang coming from the Liver and Stomach. This massage aims to regulate Qi-blood flow in the face, and to calm the flourishing Yang.

Step 1

Start treatment by opening the Channels in the head region (see pp. 47-9). Take extra point *Yintang*, Du20 (*Baihui*), extra point *Taiyang*, St6 (*Jiache*), SI19 (*Tinggong*), and GB20 (*Fengchi*) as major acupoints. Press them a few more times than other points in the sequence, for example, 30 to 40 times each.

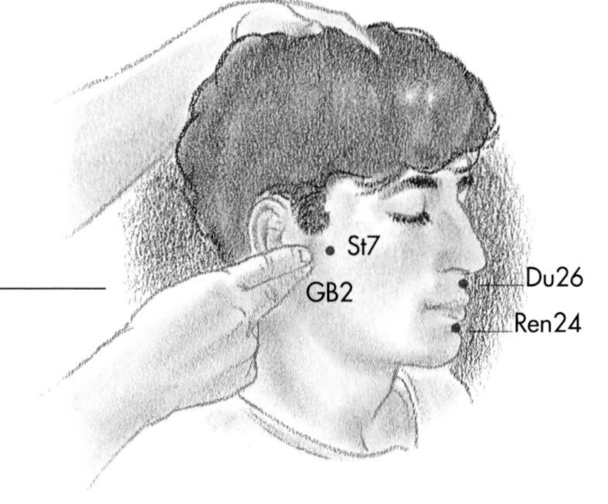

Step 2

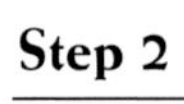

With your fingers, press acupoints St7 (*Xiaguan*) and GB2 (*Tinghui*) on the affected side. Then press Du26 (*Renzhong*) and Ren24 (*Chengjiang*). Press each point 30 times.

Step 3

With your thumb, press pain-relief point A1 firmly on one hand for three minutes. Repeat on the other hand. Then press acupoints T5 (*Waiguan*), L14 (*Hegu*), P6 (*Neiguan*), and H7 (*Shenmen*) on the affected side (or both sides). Press the points in sequence, 30 times each.

Step 4

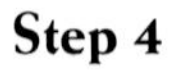

Ask your partner to lie down, face up. With both your thumbs, press acupoints Ren12 (*Zhongwan*) and Ren6 (*Qihai*) simultaneously. Repeat about 30 times.

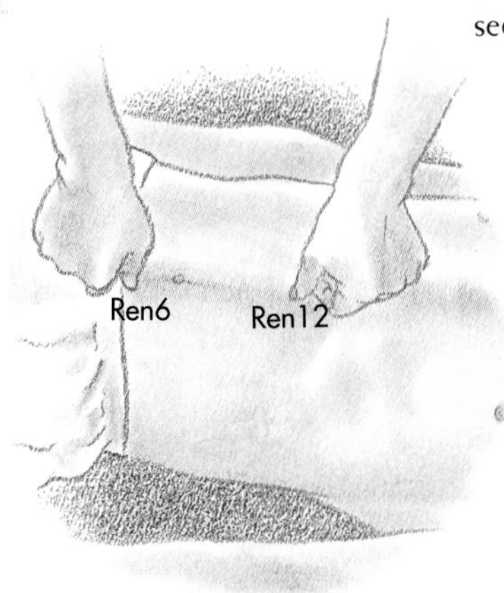

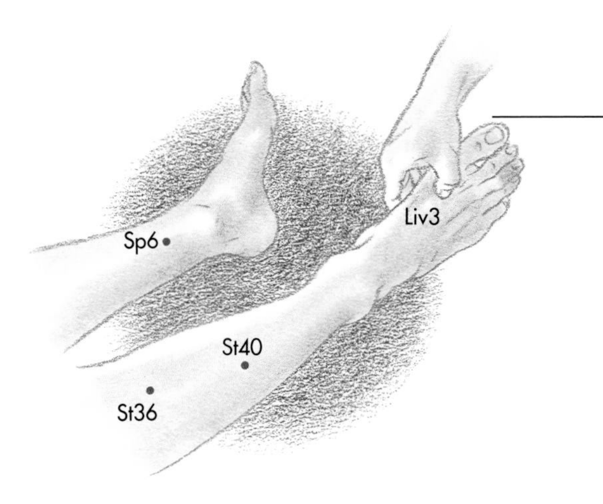

Step 5

Press acupoints St36 (*Zusanli*), St40 (*Fenglong*), Sp6 (*Sanyinjiao*), and Liv3 (*Taichong*) on the leg of the affected side (or on both sides). Use your thumb, and press each successive point 30 times.

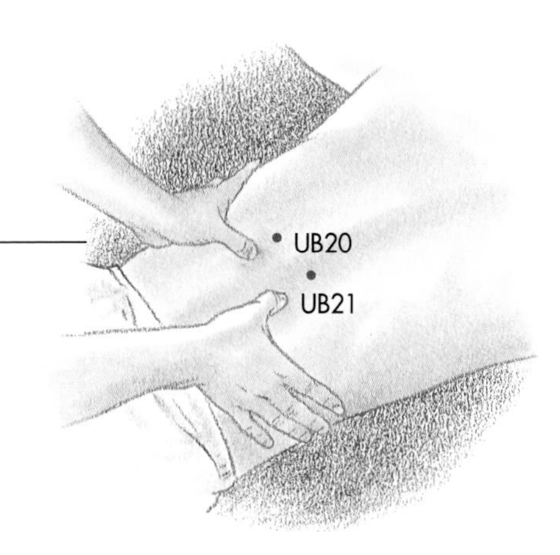

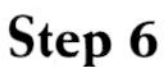

Step 6

Ask your partner to turn over and lie face down. With your thumbs, press both UB20 (*Pishu*) and both UB21 (*Weishu*) acupoints about 30 times.

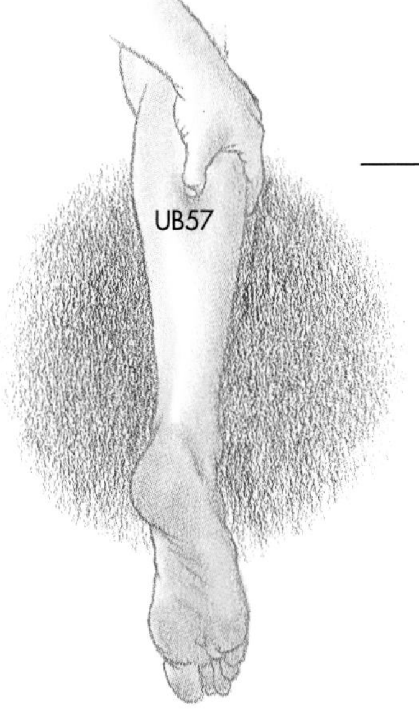

Step 7

With your thumb, press acupoint UB57 (*Chengshan*) on the leg of your partner's affected side (or on both sides) about 30 times.

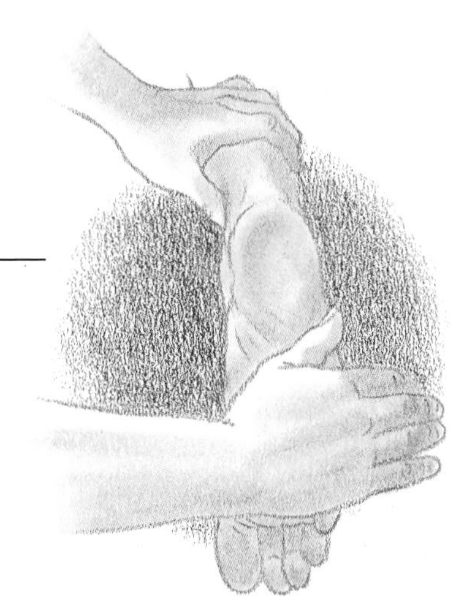

Step 8

Rub acupoint K1 (*Yongquan*) on the sole of your partner's affected side, with the heel of your hand. Rub up and down over the point until your partner feels warm there. Repeat on the other foot if necessary.

PEPTIC ULCERS AND CHRONIC GASTRITIS

These common complaints are often due to stress, or to an inappropriate diet of rich food and excessive alcohol. Both conditions cause stomachache, and a range of other symptoms that are similar to exaggerated indigestion (dyspepsia). For example, discomfort and pain after eating, loss of appetite, abdominal distension, and vomiting may all accompany the stomachache.

Pain-relief massage aims to strengthen the Stomach and Spleen, to expel negative Qi, and to reduce fullness in the Stomach. Use this treatment as a guide for treating similar conditions.

CAUTION
DO NOT MASSAGE IF YOUR PARTNER IS VOMITING BLOOD OR HAS A PERFORATED STOMACH. SEEK MEDICAL ADVICE BEFORE TREATING ACUTE GASTRITIS.

Step 1

Start treatment by opening the Channels in the abdomen (see pp. 50-3). Press acupoints Ren12 (*Zhongwan*), Ren6 (*Qihai*), Ren4 (*Guanyuan*), and both St25 (*Tianshu*) a few more times than others in the sequence, for example, 30 to 40 times each.

Step 2

Open the Channels in the back (see pp. 54-6). Take UB20 (*Pishu*), UB21 (*Weishu*), and UB23 (*Shenshu*) as the major acupoints. Press them a few more times than others in the sequence, for example, 30 to 40 times each.

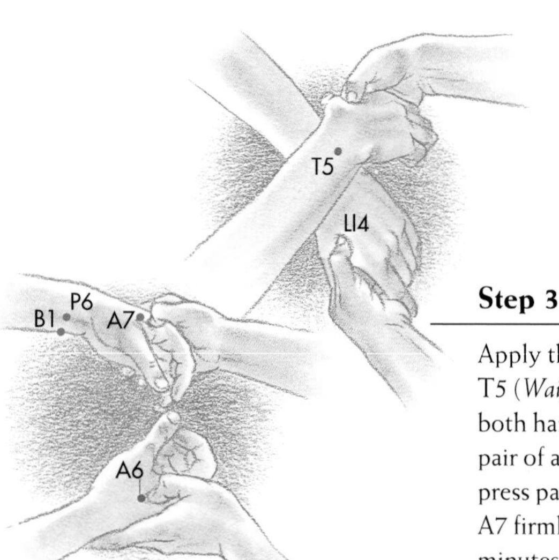

Step 3

Apply thumb pressure to LI4 (*Hegu*), T5 (*Waiguan*), and P6 (*Neiguan*) on both hands. Press each successive pair of acupoints 30 times. Then press pain-relief points B1, A6, and A7 firmly on both hands, for two minutes each.

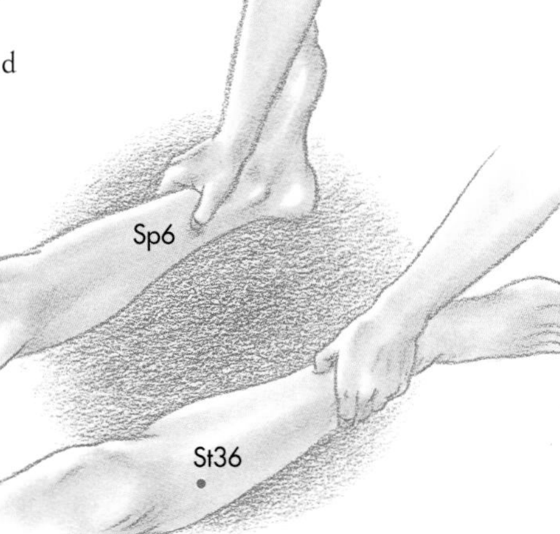

Step 4

Apply thumb pressure to acupoints St36 (*Zusanli*) and then Sp6 (*Sanyinjiao*) on both legs. Press each pair 30 to 40 times.

ACUTE ABDOMINAL PAIN

This broad description refers to irregular, sudden, and painful spasms in either the stomach or intestines, which are sometimes known as gastrospasms or enterospasms, respectively. A gastrospasm causes pain in the stomach region, while an enterospasm causes pain around the navel. Both can be caused by excessive exercise, an inappropriate diet, too much cold food, vomiting, or diarrhoea. Stomach pains may sometimes be a symptom of neurosis. Chinese medicine indicates that stomachache is caused by stagnated Qi and blood in the abdominal region. You can use the massage sequence below to treat a range of conditions that cause similar symptoms of stomachache.

CAUTION
DO NOT MASSAGE IF STOMACH PAINS ARE CAUSED BY ACUTE GASTRITIS OR INFLAMMATION OF ANY OTHER INTERNAL ORGAN, EXCEPT UNDER MEDICAL SUPERVISION.

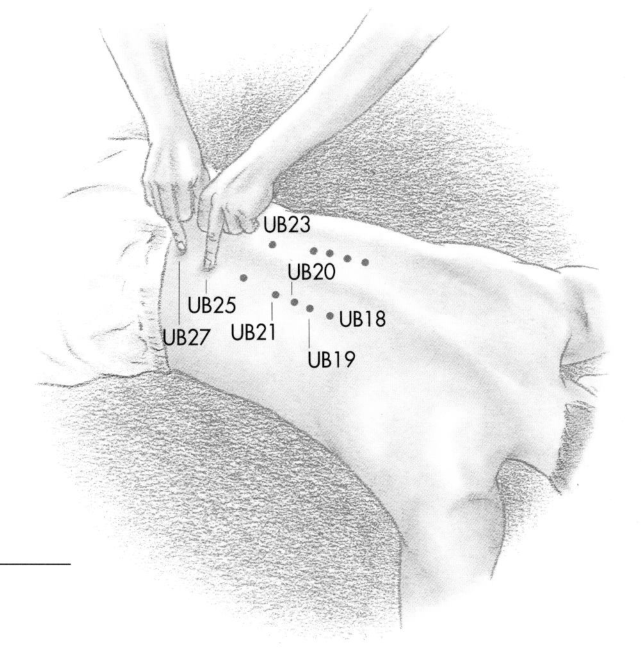

Step 1

Using your thumb and index finger, press the following pairs of acupoints either side of the spine: UB18 (*Ganshu*), UB19 (*Danshu*), UB20 (*Pishu*), UB21 (*Weishu*), UB23 (*Shenshu*), UB25 (*Dachangshu*), and UB27 (*Xiaochangshu*). Press each pair 30 times. You can, if you wish, use both hands and work on two pairs simultaneously.

Step 2

Work down the back, from top to bottom, pinching the extra points *Jiaji* either side of the spine. Repeat five times. Then, with your palm, push down the Urinary Bladder Channel on one side of the spine from top to bottom. Repeat five times. Then push down the Urinary Bladder Channel on the other side of the spine five times.

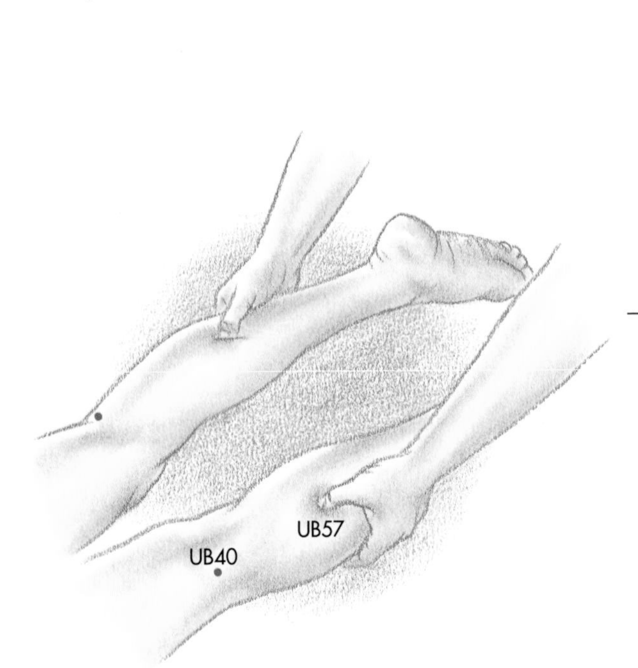

Step 3

Press acupoints UB40 (*Weizhong*) and UB57 (*Chengshan*) on both legs. Use thumb pressure, and press each pair about 30 times.

Step 4

Apply the sequence for opening the Channels in the abdomen (see pp. 50-3). Treat Ren12 (*Zhongwan*), Ren6 (*Qihai*), both St25 (*Tianshu*), and both Liv13 (*Zhangmen*) as major acupoints, and press them a few more times than others in the sequence, for example, 30 to 40 times each.

Step 5

Apply the rolling manipulation to the affected part of the abdomen for about one minute (see also p. 41).

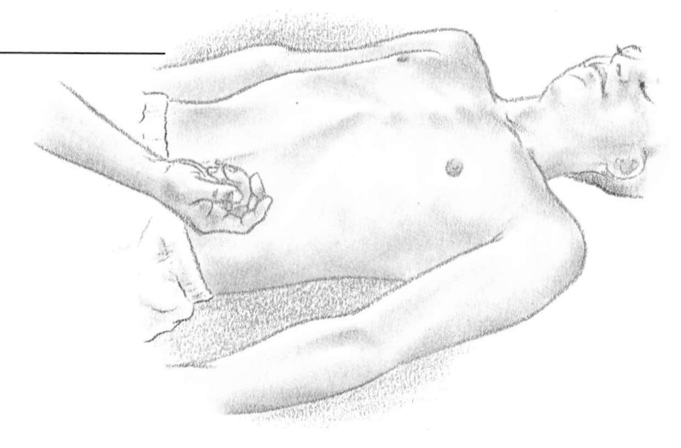

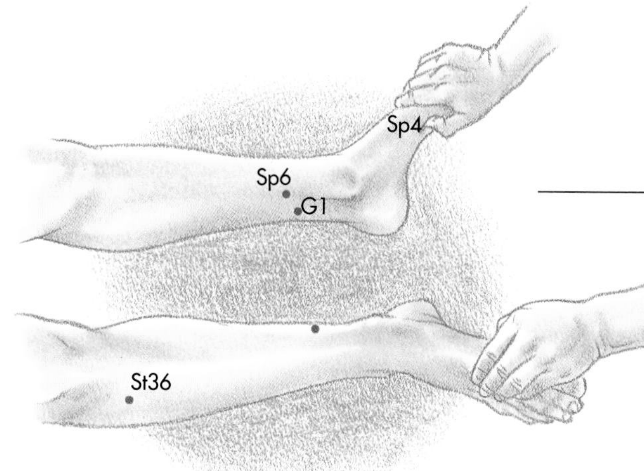

Step 6

With your thumbs, press acupoints St36 (*Zusanli*), Sp6 (*Sanyinjiao*), Sp4 (*Gongsun*), and pain-relief point G1 on both legs. Press one pair of points at a time, about 30 times.

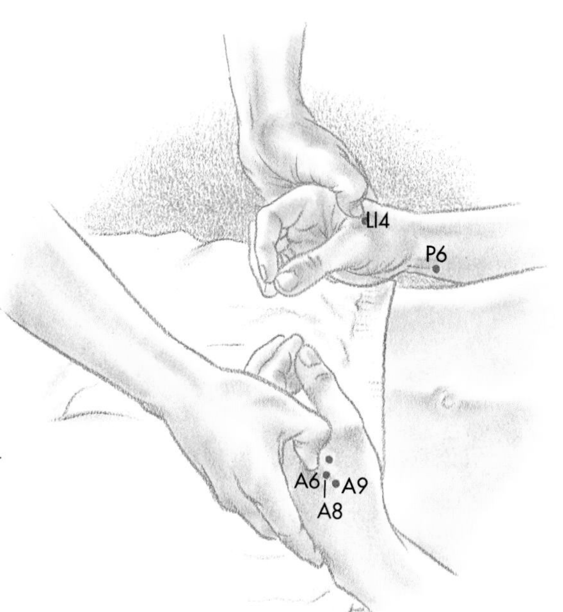

Step 7

Press acupoints LI4 (*Hegu*) and P6 (*Neiguan*) about 30 times each on both hands. Then press pain-relief points A6, A8, and A9 on both hands, for about two minutes each.

GALL BLADDER PAIN

Gall bladder pain is often caused by gallstones, which can form in the gall bladder from an excessive concentration of bile, notably cholesterol, and can cause great pain. The gall bladder can also become inflamed, a condition known as chronic cholecystitis. Inflammation causes abdominal pain, as well as indigestion, nausea, and flatulence, especially after eating a fatty meal.

CAUTION
JAUNDICE (YELLOW SKIN COLOUR AND EYES) MAY INDICATE A BLOCKAGE BY A GALLSTONE. SEEK IMMEDIATE MEDICAL ATTENTION.

Step 1

Start the pain-relief massage by opening the Channels in the abdominal region (see pp. 50-3).

Step 2

Using your thumbs, press acupoint P6 (*Neiguan*) on both hands about 30 times. Then press both A5 pain-relief points for two minutes.

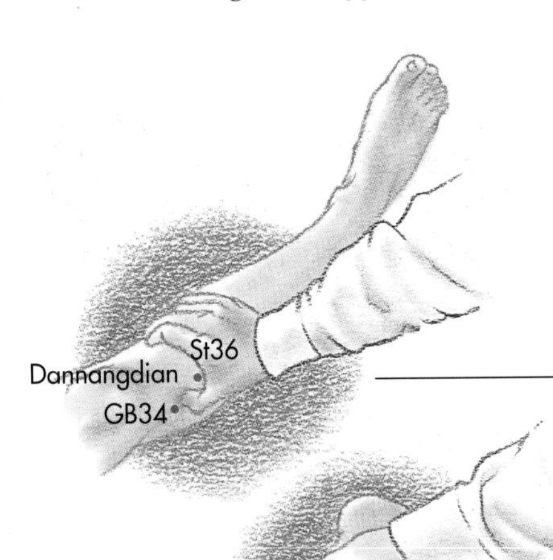

Step 3

With your thumbs press GB34 (*Yanglingquan*), extra point *Dannangdian*, St36 (*Zusanli*), and pain-relief points G1 and G2 on the affected side or on both legs. Press each point about 30 times, except *Dannangdian*, which you should press firmly for three minutes.

Step 4

Ask your partner to turn over, and lie face down. With your thumbs and index fingers, press both UB18 (*Ganshu*) and both UB19 (*Danshu*) acupoints simultaneously. Repeat 40 to 50 times.

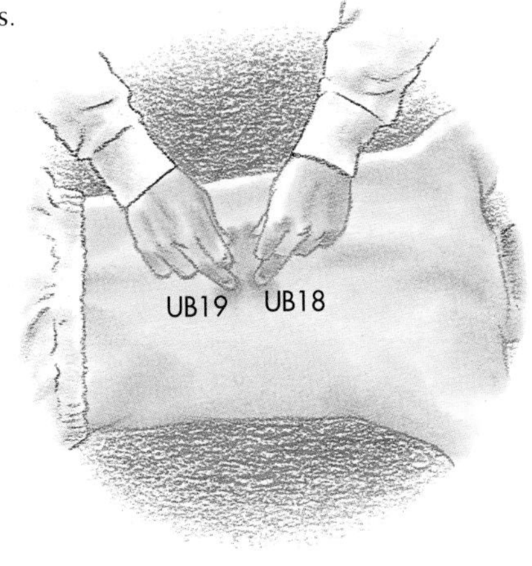

CONSTIPATION

Constipation commonly results from a lack of fibre in the diet. However, a lack of physical exercise, stress, and emotional factors can also be to blame. The stools are dark, hard, and difficult to pass. In severe cases, the abdomen may swell from the remnants of digestion.

According to Chinese medicine, constipation often results from a deficiency of Qi, a weakness of Yang, or stagnated Qi. Together these conditions have a negative effect on the functions of the Large Intestine. Massage can make up the Qi deficiency, and remove the stagnation. A spoonful of honey taken 10 minutes before breakfast every day will also help to treat constipation.

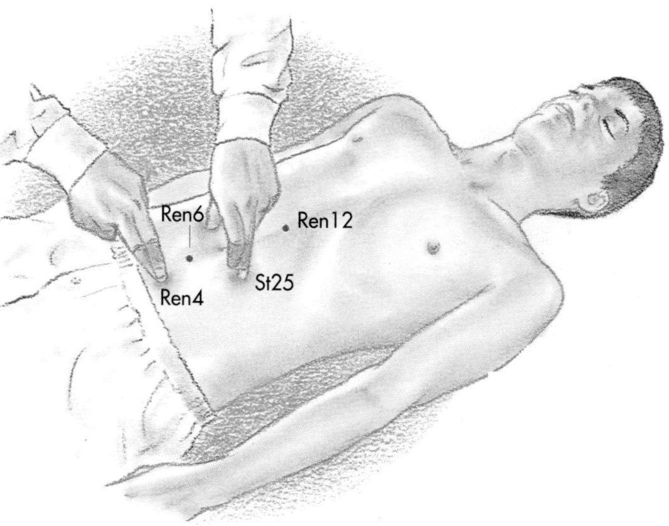

Step 1

Use finger pressure to press Ren12 (*Zhongwan*), both St25 (*Tianshu*), Ren6 (*Qihai*), and Ren4 (*Guanyuan*) acupoints. Press each point about 30 times, except for St25, which you should press 40 to 50 times. If you wish, you can press two sets of points simultaneously.

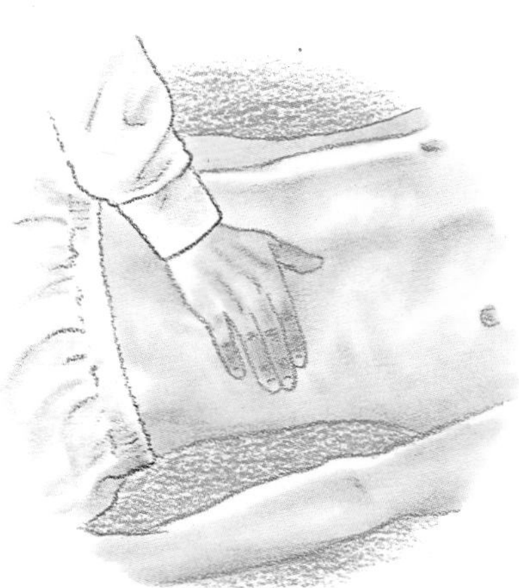

Step 2

Press and knead the navel with the heel of your hand. Then rub around the navel with your palm until the area feels warm to your partner.

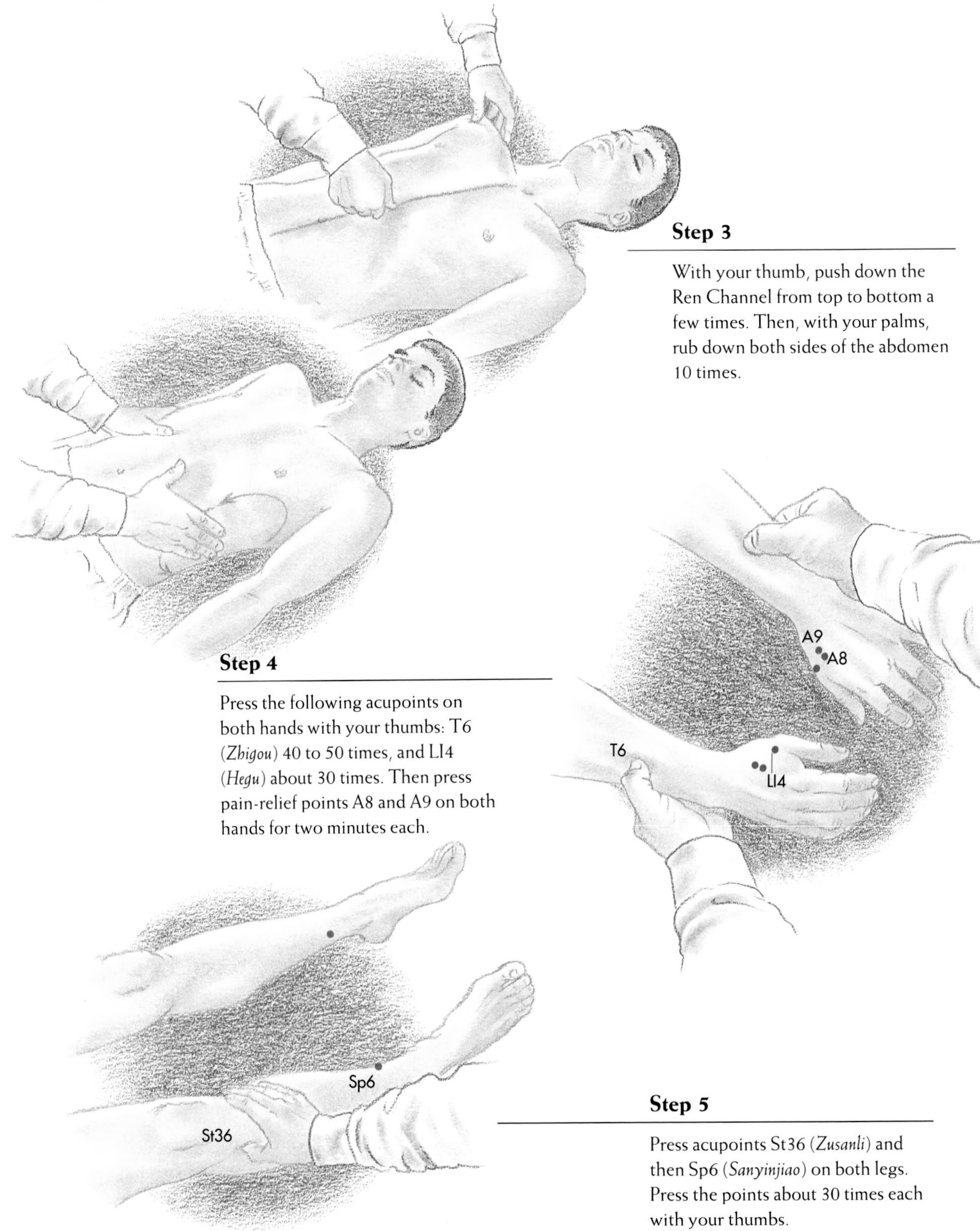

Step 3

With your thumb, push down the Ren Channel from top to bottom a few times. Then, with your palms, rub down both sides of the abdomen 10 times.

Step 4

Press the following acupoints on both hands with your thumbs: T6 (*Zhigou*) 40 to 50 times, and LI4 (*Hegu*) about 30 times. Then press pain-relief points A8 and A9 on both hands for two minutes each.

Step 5

Press acupoints St36 (*Zusanli*) and then Sp6 (*Sanyinjiao*) on both legs. Press the points about 30 times each with your thumbs.

Step 6

Press the following acupoints in their pairs on either side of the spine: UB20 (*Pishu*), UB21 (*Weishu*), UB23 (*Shenshu*), UB25 (*Dachangshu*), and UB27 (*Xiaochangshu*). Press each pair 30 to 40 times, with your thumbs.

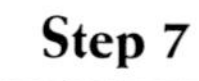

Step 7

Percuss acupoints UB31-34 (*Baliao*) with a loosely clenched fist 20 times (see also p. 43). Then rub the area with your palm until it feels warm to your partner.

Step 8

With your thumbs, press acupoint UB57 (*Chengshan*) on both legs 30 to 40 times.

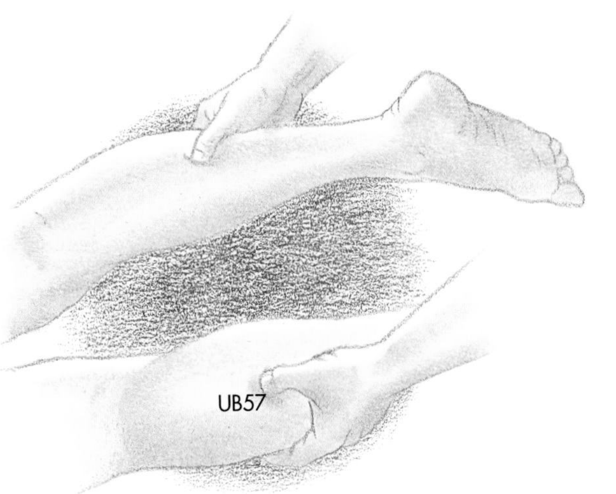

CHRONIC PELVIC INFLAMMATION

This disease is usually caused when an infection of the vagina or another nearby organ spreads to, and inflames, the female reproductive organs. Symptoms include pain and fullness in the lower abdomen, and soreness in the lower back. Tiredness, insomnia, dizziness, and loss of appetite may also be present. Chronic pelvic inflammation often results from untreated acute pelvic inflammation. Pain-relief massage aims to strengthen the Spleen and the Kidneys, to regulate Qi, and to expel Cold (see p. 9), which often causes the problem.

CAUTION
DO NOT APPLY PAIN-RELIEF MASSAGE FOR ACUTE PELVIC INFLAMMATION UNLESS UNDER MEDICAL SUPERVISION.

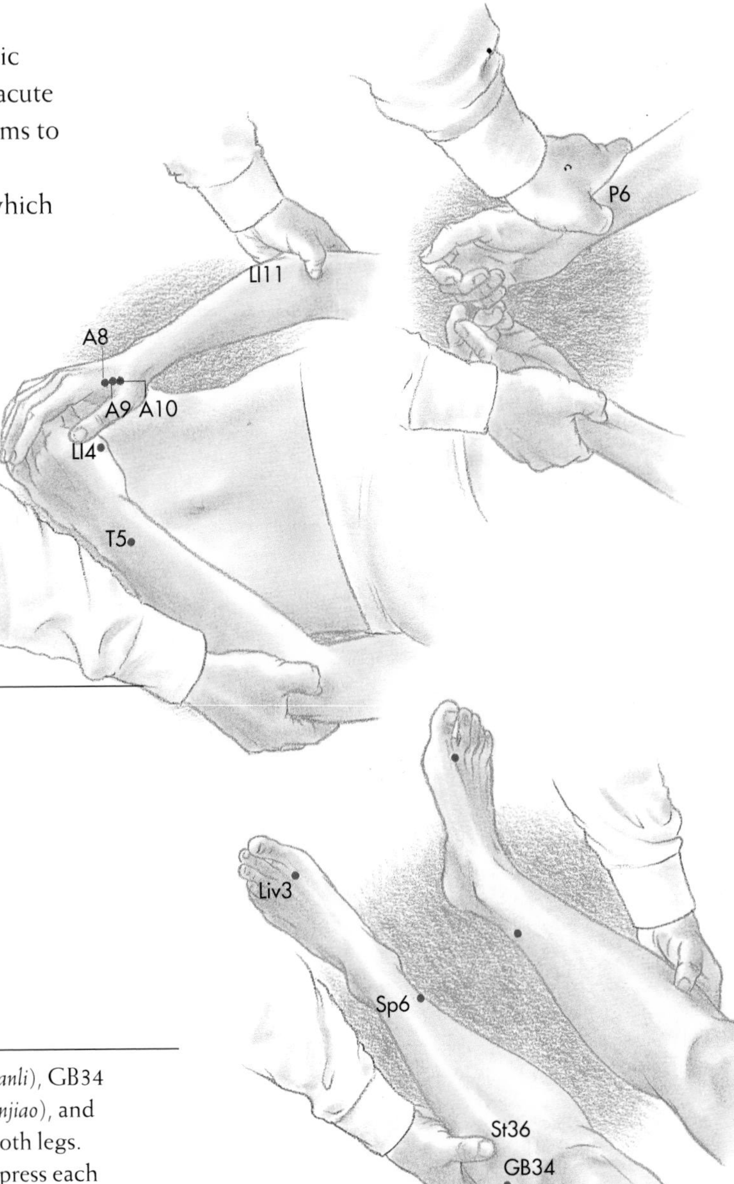

Step 1

Open the Channels in the abdomen (see pp. 50-3), taking Ren12 (*Zhongwan*), both Liv13 (*Zhangmen*), Ren6 (*Qihai*), and Ren4 (*Guanyuan*) as the major acupoints. Press them a few more times each than the other points, for example, 30 to 40 times.

Step 2

With your thumbs, press acupoints P6 (*Neiguan*), LI11 (*Quchi*), T5 (*Waiguan*), and LI4 (*Hegu*) in succession. Press the points on both arms about 30 times each. Then press pain-relief points A8, A9, and A10 on both hands, for two minutes each.

Step 3

Press acupoints St36 (*Zusanli*), GB34 (*Yanglingquan*), Sp6 (*Sanyinjiao*), and then Liv3 (*Taichong*), on both legs. Use thumb pressure, and press each pair of points about 30 times.

Step 4

Using your palm, rub the lower abdomen. Then rub the inside of the right thigh, until it feels warm to your partner. Repeat on the left thigh.

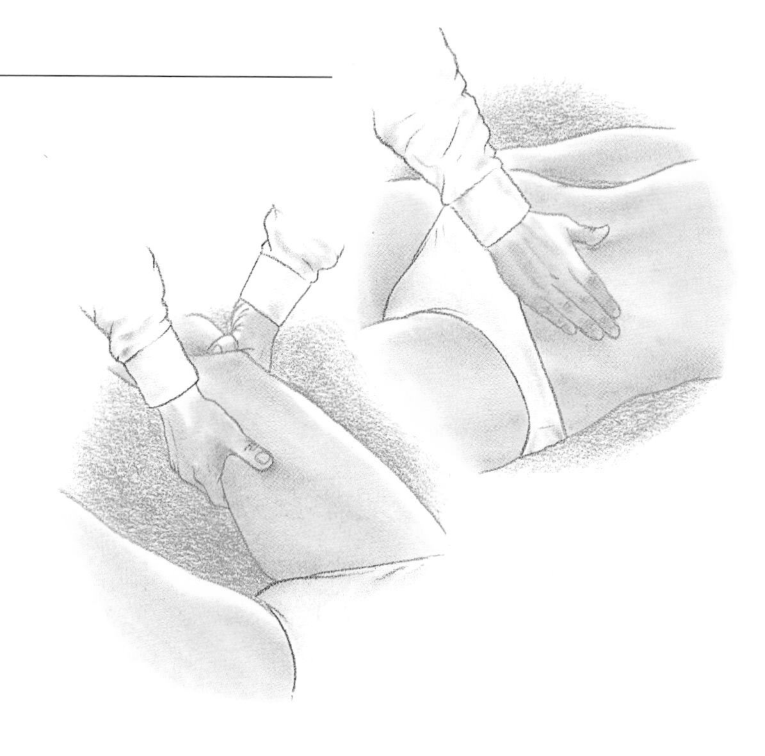

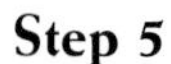

Step 5

Perform the sequence for opening the Channels in the back region (see pp. 54-6). Take UB18 (*Ganshu*), UB20 (*Pishu*), UB23 (*Shenshu*), and UB31-34 (*Baliao*) as the major acupoints, pressing them a few more times than others in the sequence, for example, 30 to 40 times each.

Step 6

Using your palm, rub the lower back. Continue rubbing until it feels warm to your partner.

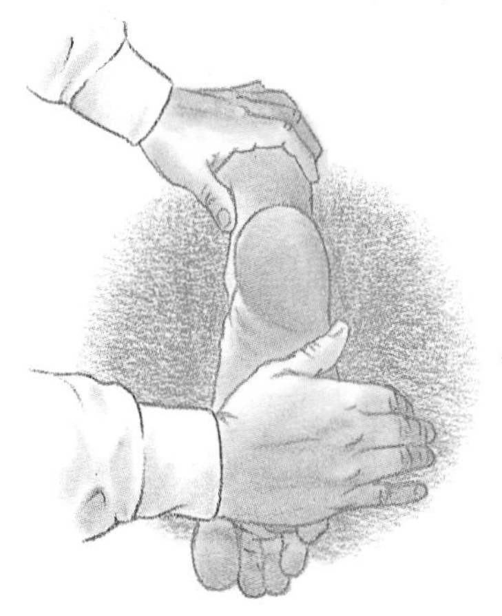

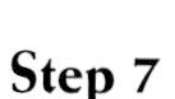

Step 7

Using the heel of your hand, rub up and down over acupoint K1 (*Yongquan*) on the sole of the right foot until it is warm. Repeat on the left foot.

PERIOD PAIN

Period pain, or dysmenorrhoea, affects a great many women immediately prior to, or during, bleeding. The pain may range from a slight discomfort to intensely painful cramps in the lower abdomen, or the lower back. Typically, period pains are caused by anaemia, hormonal imbalances, chills and exhaustion, or inflammation of the reproductive organs.

Chinese medicine indicates that painful periods result from stagnated Qi, blood stasis, a deficiency of Qi and blood, or a weakness of the Liver and Kidneys. Massage strengthens the Liver and Kidneys, and clears the Channel blockage. Ideally, you should start massage one week before your partner's period is due.

UB18
Du4
UB20
UB23

Step 1

Press acupoints UB18 (*Ganshu*), UB20 (*Pishu*), and then UB23 (*Shenshu*), in pairs on either side of the spine. Then press Du4 (*Mingmen*). Press the points 30 times each with your thumbs.

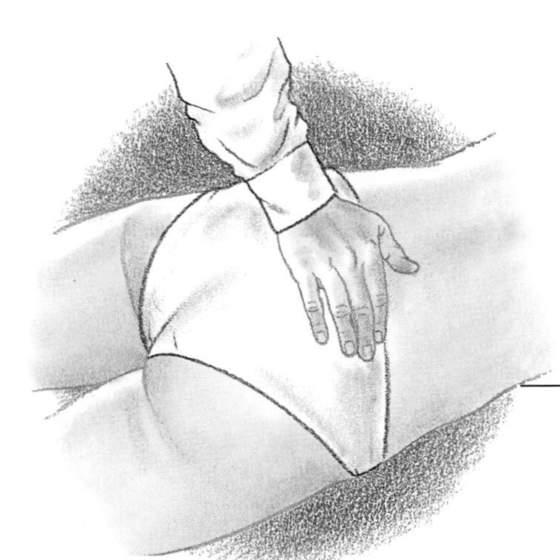

Step 2

Rub acupoints UB31-34 (*Baliao*) with the heel of your hand. Continue rubbing until the area feels warm to your partner.

Step 3

Push down the Du Channel with the heel of your hand. Repeat five times. Then push down both Urinary Bladder Channels either side of the spine. Repeat five times for each Channel.

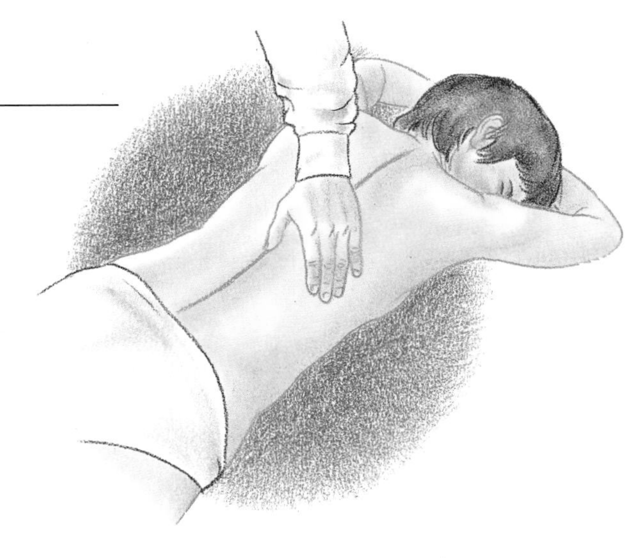

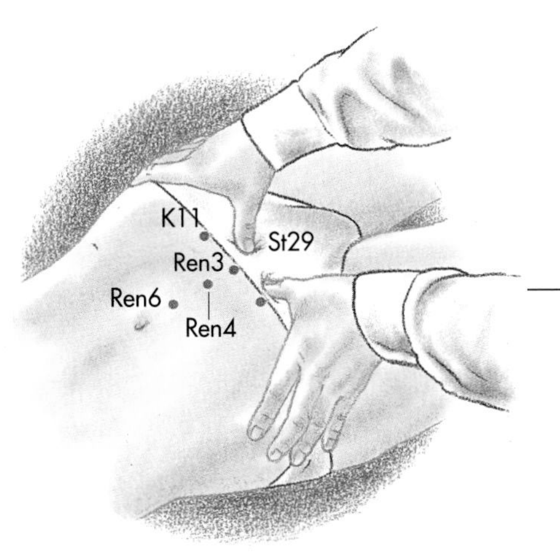

Step 4

Press and knead Ren6 (*Qihai*), Ren4 (*Guanyuan*), Ren3 (*Zhongji*), both St29 (*Guilai*), and both K11 (*Henggu*) acupoints in succession. Press each point 30 times with your thumbs.

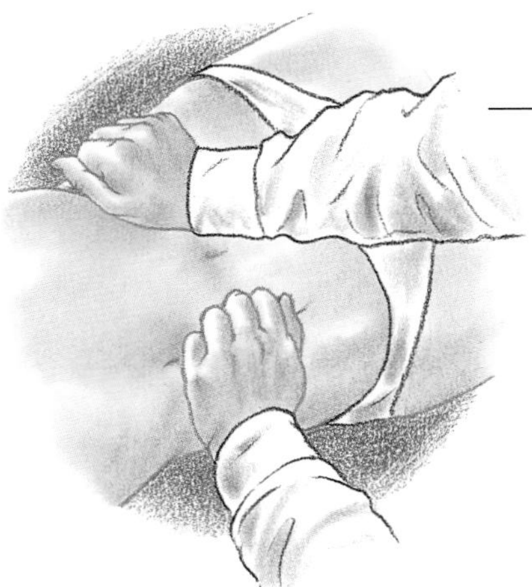

Step 5

Squeeze acupoint GB26 (*Daimai*) on both sides of the abdomen. Fold the points over the abdomen, and then release. Repeat three times.

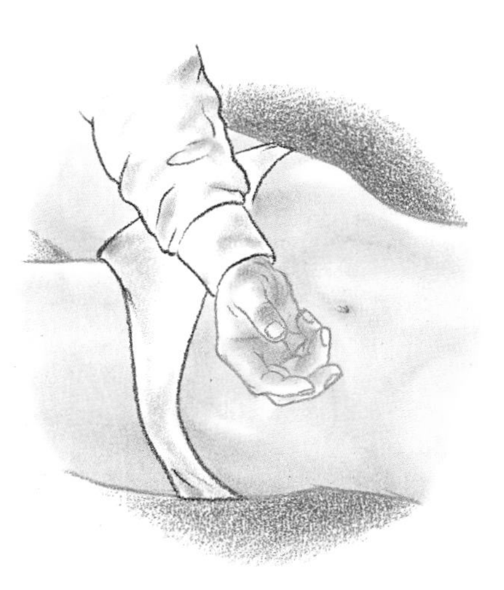

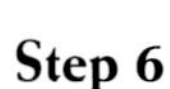

Step 6

Rub around your partner's navel with your palm. Then roll the side of your hand backward and forward over the lower abdomen (see right). Your hand should be curled as you apply the rolling massage (see also p. 41).

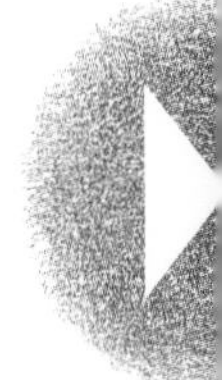

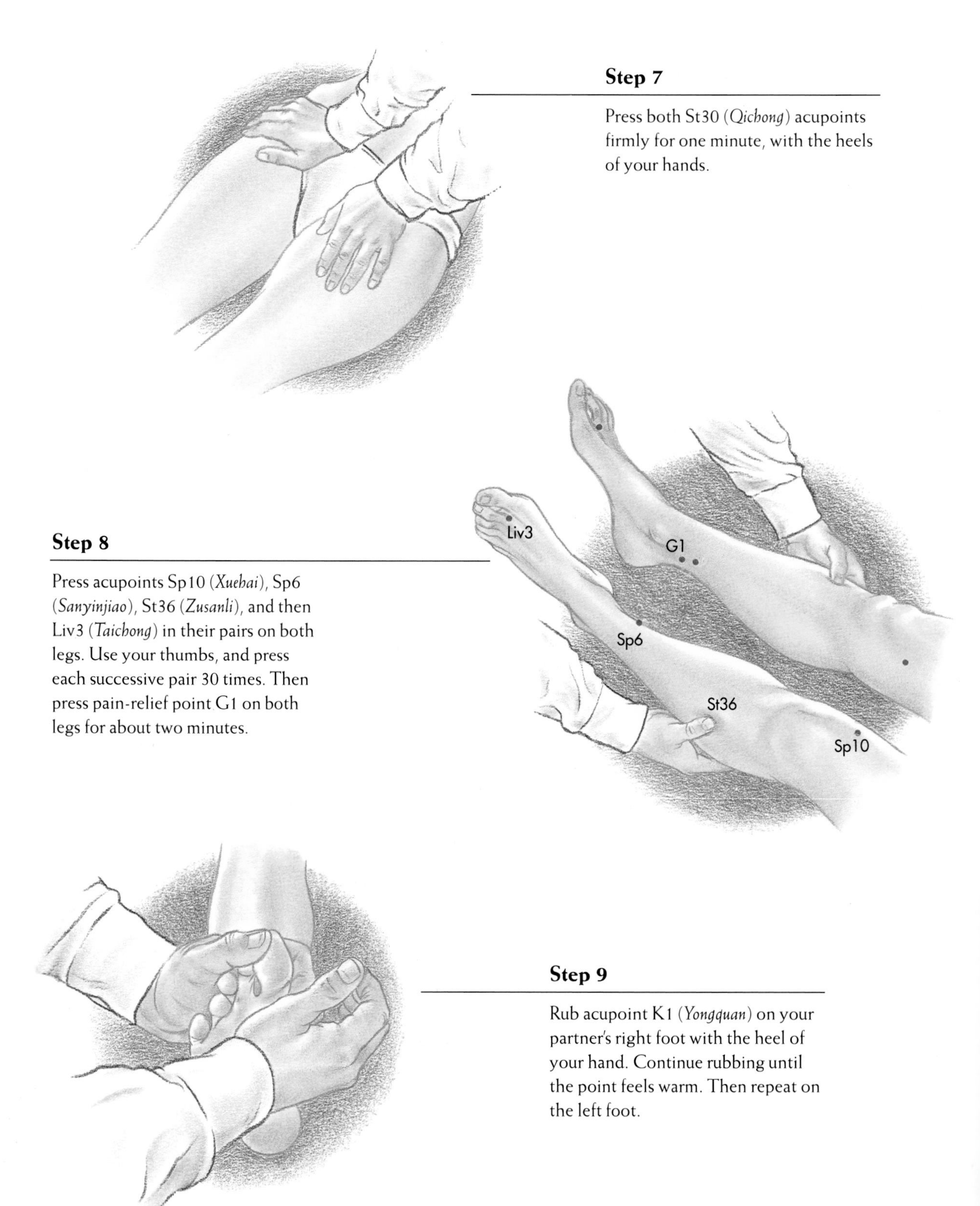

Step 7

Press both St30 (*Qichong*) acupoints firmly for one minute, with the heels of your hands.

Step 8

Press acupoints Sp10 (*Xuehai*), Sp6 (*Sanyinjiao*), St36 (*Zusanli*), and then Liv3 (*Taichong*) in their pairs on both legs. Use your thumbs, and press each successive pair 30 times. Then press pain-relief point G1 on both legs for about two minutes.

Step 9

Rub acupoint K1 (*Yongquan*) on your partner's right foot with the heel of your hand. Continue rubbing until the point feels warm. Then repeat on the left foot.

INTERCOSTAL NEURALGIA

Intercostal neuralgia affects the nerves that run from the spine through the spaces between the ribs to the front of the body. Some localized areas, where the affected nerve reaches the skin, may be particularly painful.

In Chinese medicine, this disorder is simply called rib pain. It is thought to be due to depressed Qi in the Liver. The massage steps below ease this depression. The affected areas on your partner's abdomen and back may be particularly tender to the touch, so be very gentle with your massage.

CAUTION
DO NOT MASSAGE IF THE INTERCOSTAL NEURALGIA IS CAUSED BY PRESSURE OR IRRITATION FROM A TUMOUR OR FROM TUBERCULOSIS.

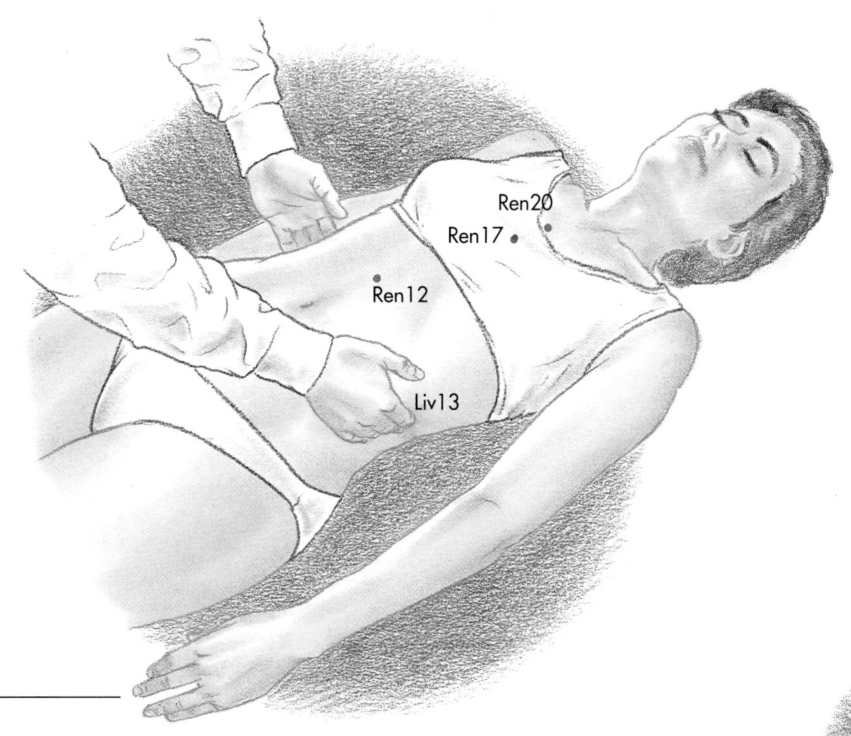

Step 1

Press Ren20 (*Huagai*), Ren17 (*Tanzhong*), Ren12 (*Zhongwan*), and both Liv13 (*Zhangmen*) acupoints in succession. Press each point 30 to 40 times.

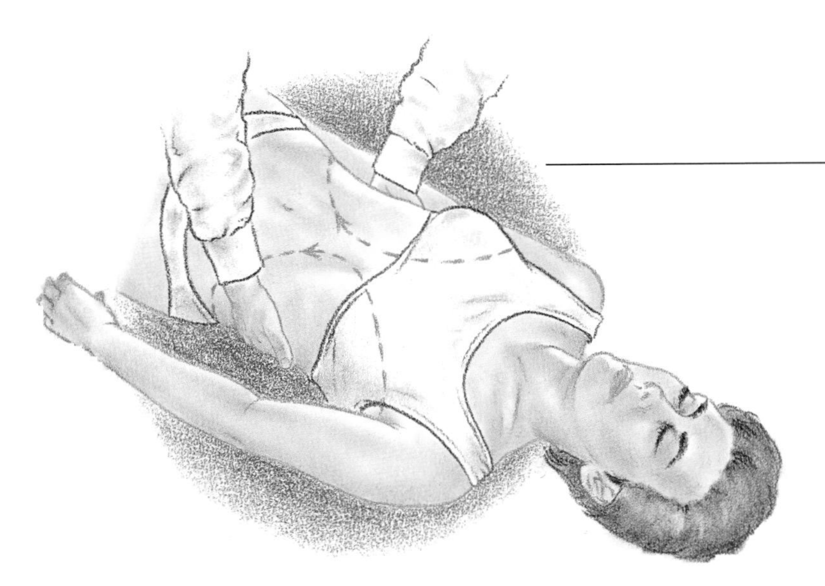

Step 2

Rub up and down over the upper part of your partner's trunk with your palms. Repeat seven times.

Step 3

Press the following acupoints in pairs on both arms: LI11 (*Quchi*), T6 (*Zhigou*), T5 (*Waiguan*), and LI4 (*Hegu*). Use your thumbs, and press each pair about 30 times. Press pain-relief point A4 on both hands for three minutes. Then press both P6 (*Neiguan*) and both P8 (*Laogong*) acupoints about 30 times each.

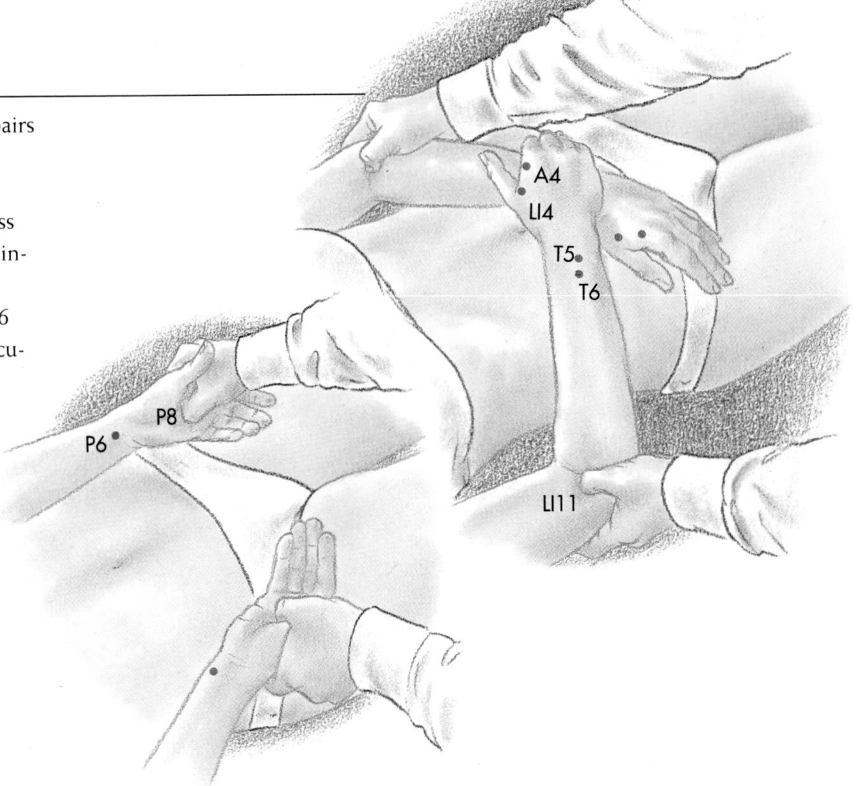

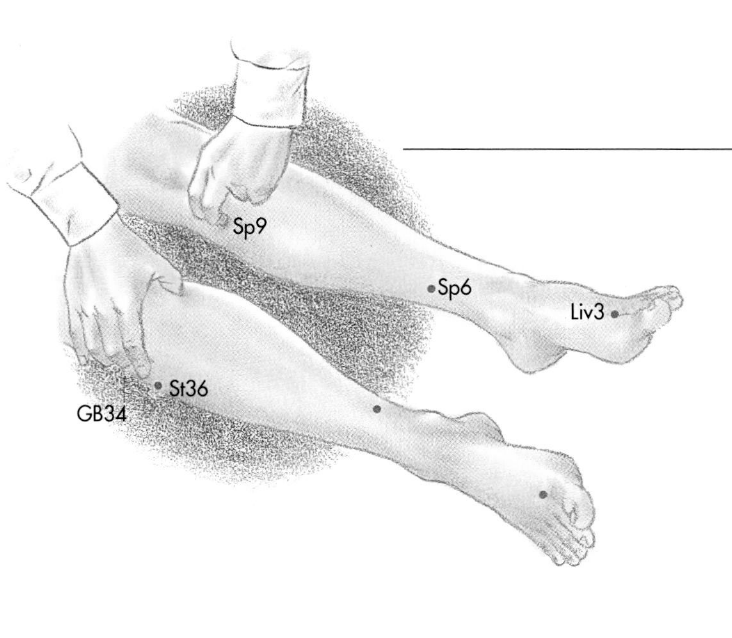

Step 4

Press Sp9 (*Yinlingquan*) and GB34 (*Yanglingquan*) acupoints simulatneously on both legs. Then press St36 (*Zusanli*), Sp6 (*Sanyinjiao*), and Liv3 (*Taichong*) in succession on both legs. Press each pair about 30 times with your thumbs.

Step 5

Open the Channels in the back region (see pp. 54-6). Press Du14 (*Dazhui*), and squeeze GB21 (*Jianjing*) a few more times than the other acupoints in the sequence, for example, 30 to 40 times each.

Step 6

Work down both sides of the spine, from the 1st thoracic to the 12th thoracic vertebra, pinching extra points *Jiaji*. Repeat 20 times.

Step 7

Rub and press the upper part of your partner's back with both palms. Pay particular attention to the painful areas, and keep massaging until the area feels warm to your partner.

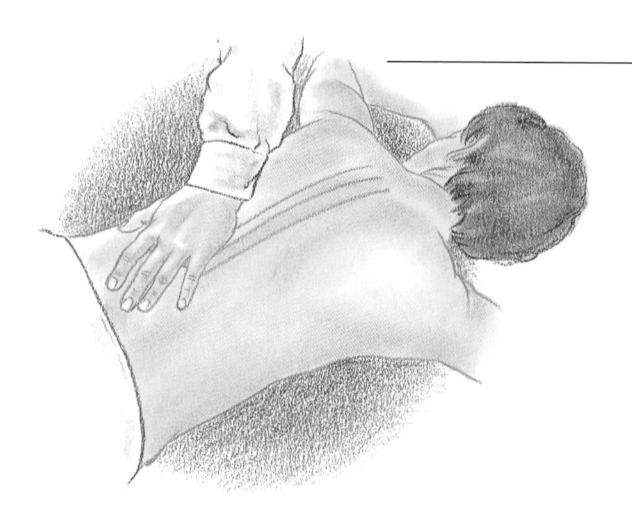

Step 8

Push down and press the spine with heel of your hand. Then do the same to the Urinary Bladder Channels that run either side of the spine. Repeat five times for each Channel.

Step 9

Percuss your partner's back with a loosely clenched fist (see also p. 43). Then tap the back with your palm for one minute (see also p. 42).

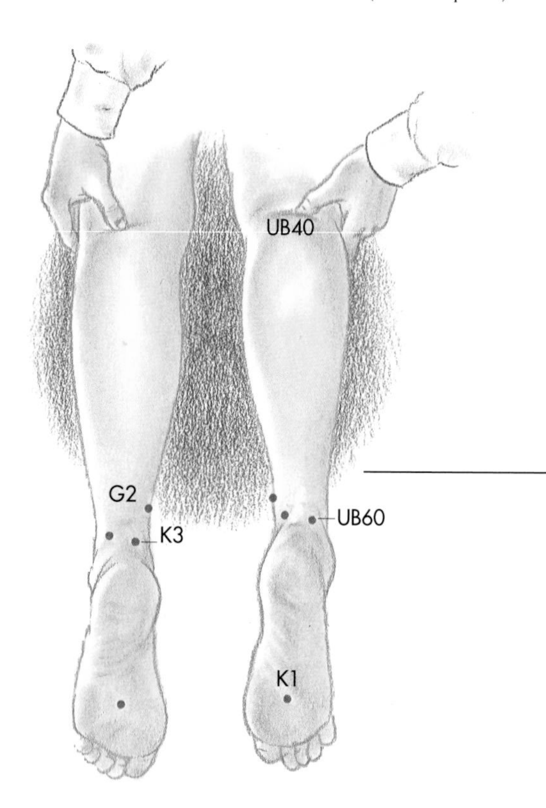

Step 10

Press acupoints UB40 (*Weizhong*), K3 (*Taixi*), UB60 (*Kunlun*), and K1 (*Yongquan*) in pairs on both legs. Press each pair 30 times with your thumbs. Then press pain-relief point G2 on both legs for about two minutes.

STIFF NECK

At times of stress, tension builds up in the neck and shoulders, causing stiffness and discomfort. A stiff neck may also be caused by sleeping in an awkward position, exposure to a cold draft, or from straining the neck muscles.

Chinese medicine suggests that a stiff neck is a symptom of Wind and Cold invading the Channels (see p. 9), causing spasms in the Channels and tendons, and a Qi-blood flow imbalance in the neck. Pain-relief massage redresses the imbalance between Qi and blood. For further improvement, apply a hot compress to the affected area after massage (see p. 30).

CAUTION
IF NECK PAIN IS CAUSED BY CERVICAL SPONDYLOSIS, SEEK MEDICAL ADVICE BEFORE TREATING WITH MASSAGE.

Step 1

Your partner should sit in a comfortable chair for this massage. With your palms, rub the neck and the upper back area to encourage your partner to relax.

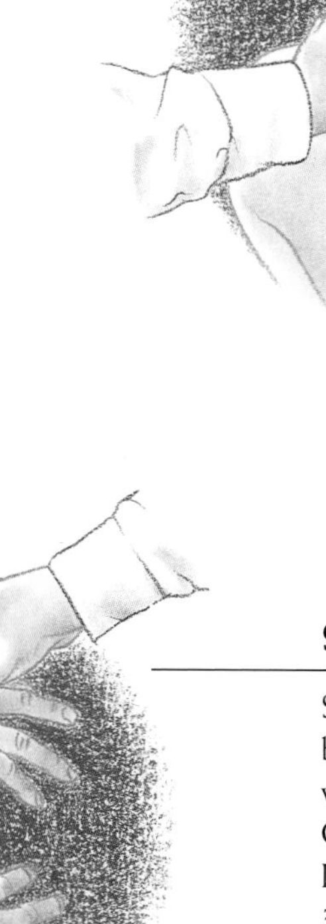

Step 2

Squeeze acupoint GB21 (*Jianjing*) on both shoulders several times. Then, with your thumbs, press acupoints GB20 (*Fengchi*), T5 (*Waiguan*), and LI4 (*Hegu*) on both sides of the body 30 times each. Then press pain-relief points A2, B6, and D on both hands for three minutes each. As you press point D, your partner should rock his or her head from side to side slowly.

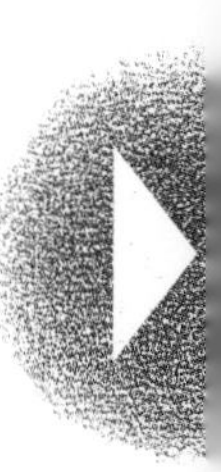

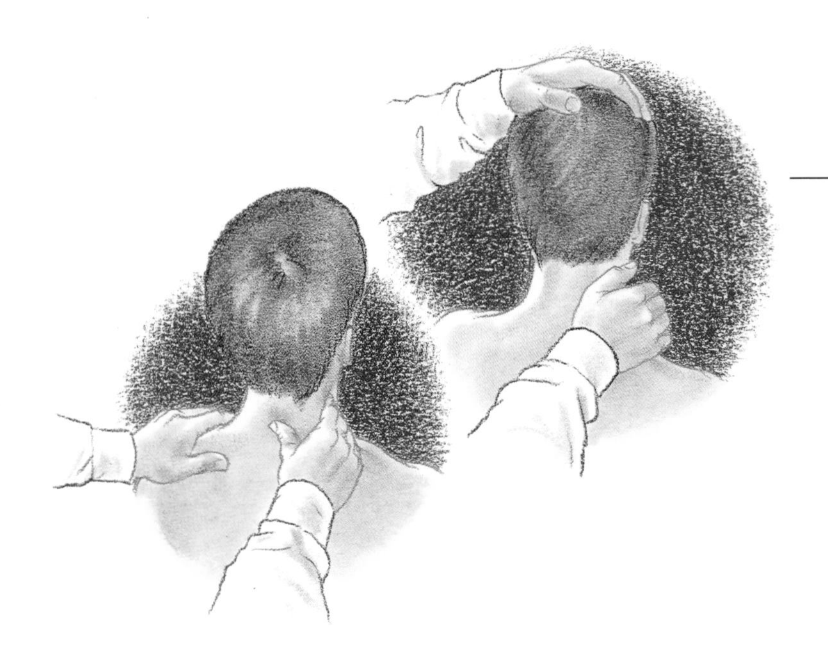

Step 3

Press and knead the pain-pressure point with the heel of your hand. Then squeeze and rub the affected area, and the neck and shoulder muscles with surgical spirits (see p. 31). Continue massaging until the muscles feel soft and warm.

Step 4

Support your partner's head by holding it under the chin and at the back of the head. Raise the head slightly, then slowly and gently turn it from side to side several times.

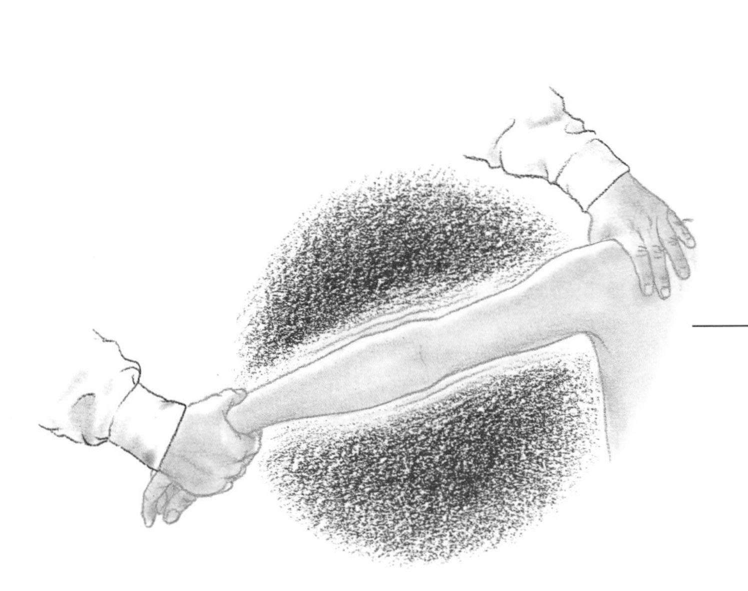

Step 5

Support your partner's right arm at the shoulder and wrist. Then gently shake the arm up and down ten times (see also p. 44). Repeat on the left arm ten times. Then squeeze both GB21 (*Jianjing*) acupoints again, as in Step 2 (see p. 93).

ACUTE BACK PAIN

Acute backache, or lumbar strain, tends to occur suddenly. For example, it may happen after carrying something very heavy or twisting awkwardly, or after working with a bad posture.

Massage is very effective in relieving back pain. It strengthens the back, reinforces the Kidneys, improves Qi-blood flow, and expels Cold and Damp (see p. 9). After massage, apply a hot compress to the affected area to further reduce the pain (see p. 30).

CAUTION
WAIT 48 HOURS AFTER INJURY OR STRAIN BEFORE YOU APPLY PAIN-RELIEF MASSAGE.

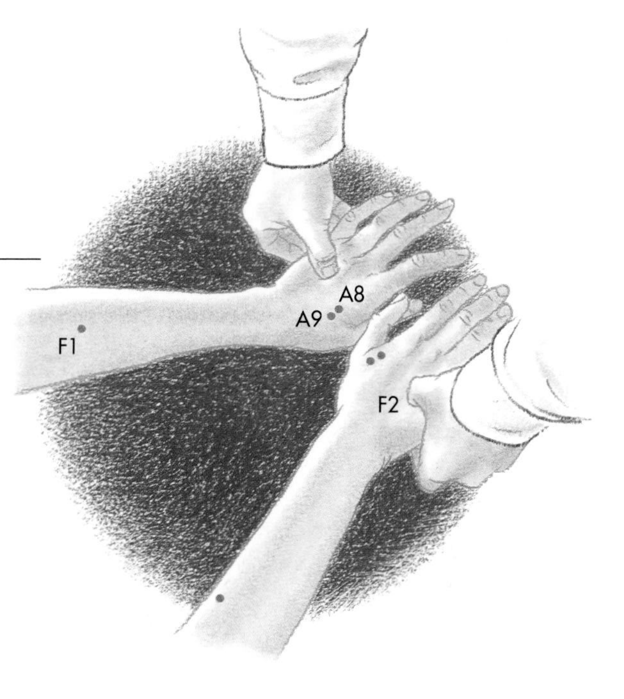

Step 1

Press pain-relief points F1, F2, A8, and A9 on both hands. Use firm thumb pressure, and press each pair for two to three minutes.

Step 2

With your whole hand, rub the painful part of the back. Use smooth, expansive, rubbing strokes to relax the back muscles.

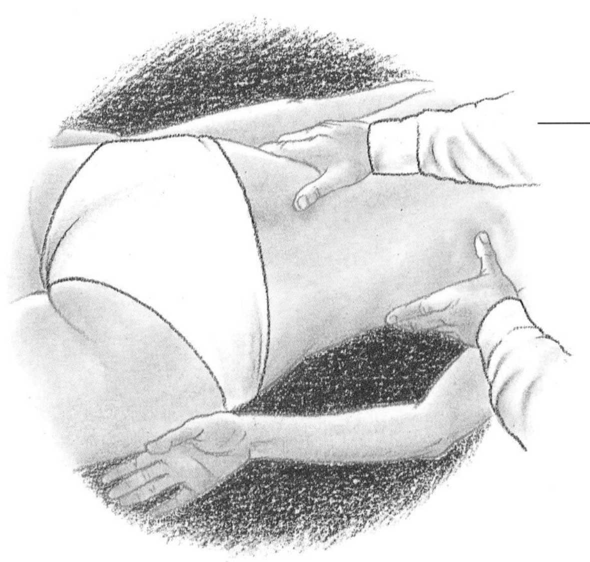

Step 3

With your palm, press and push the muscles in the painful part of the back and nearby. Apply surgical spirits to improve the effect of the massage (see p. 31). Continue rubbing until the area feels warm and comfortable to your partner.

Step 4

Press and knead the pain-pressure point with the heel of your hand. Use surgical spirits to improve the effect of the massage (see p. 31). Continue massaging until the area feels warm and comfortable to your partner.

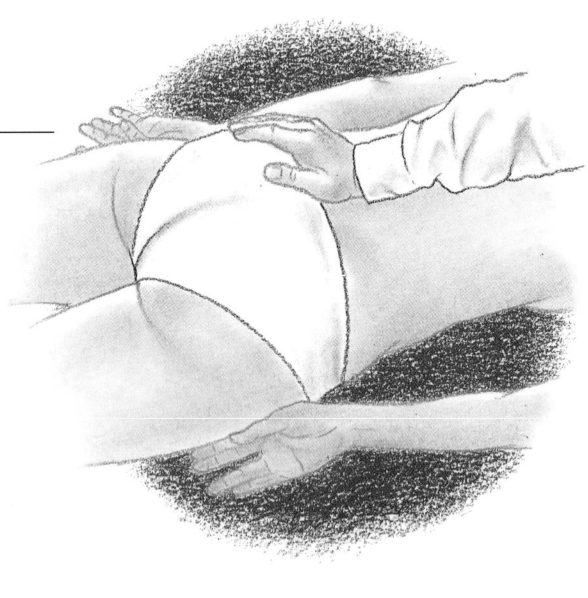

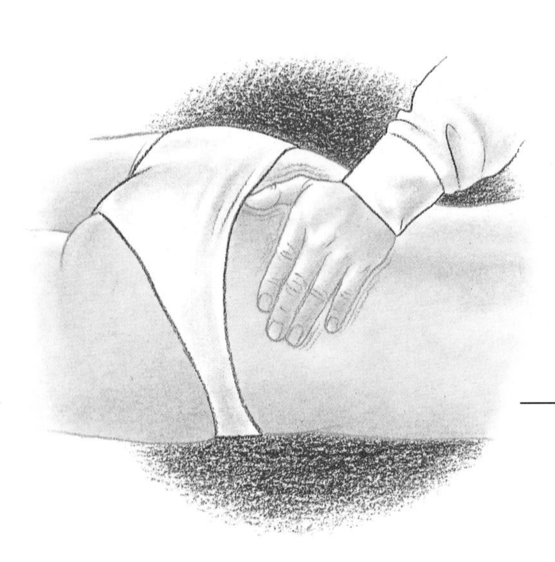

Step 5

Place your hand on the affected part of the back, and apply the quiver manipulation for about one minute (see also p. 41).

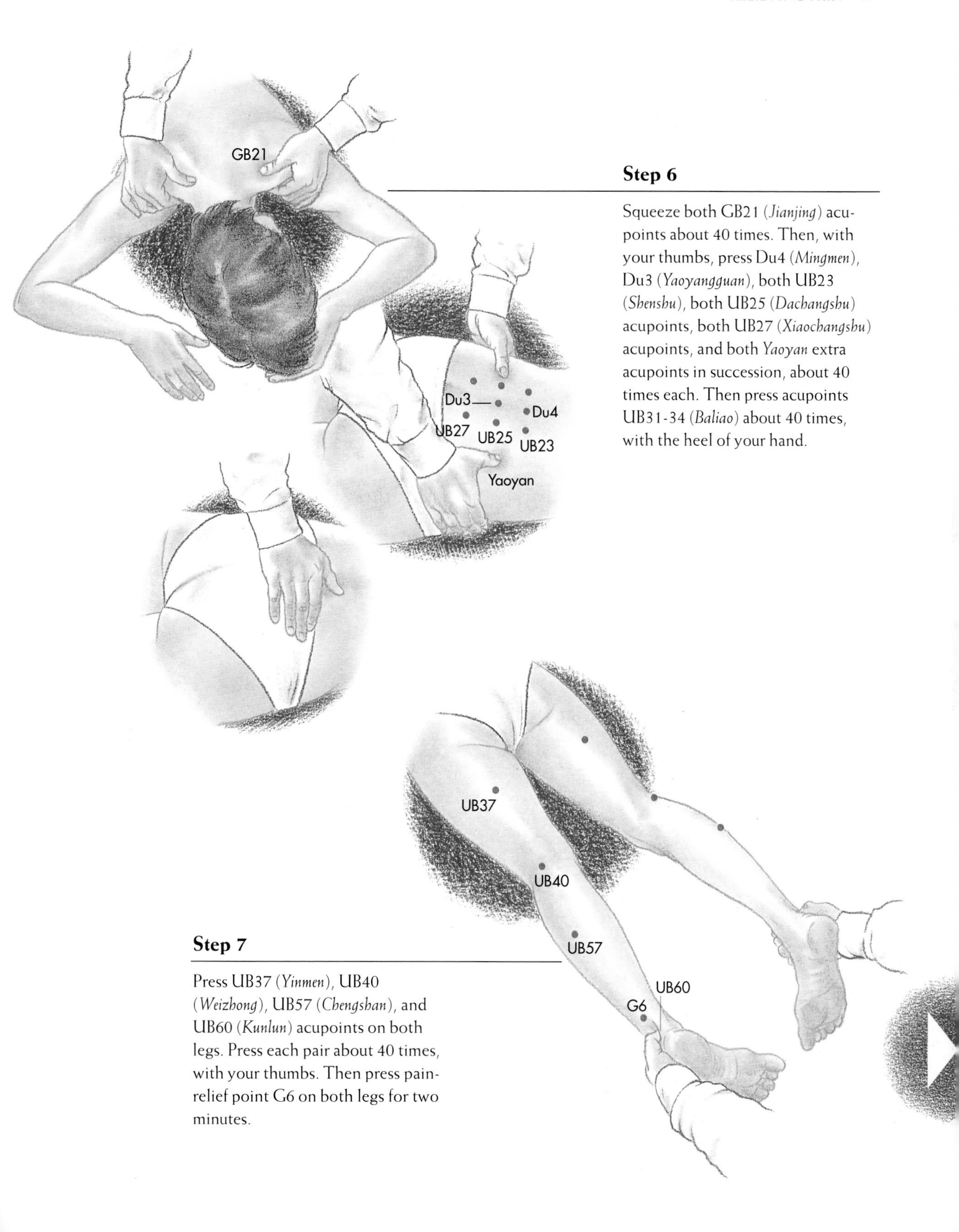

Step 6

Squeeze both GB21 (*Jianjing*) acupoints about 40 times. Then, with your thumbs, press Du4 (*Mingmen*), Du3 (*Yaoyangguan*), both UB23 (*Shenshu*), both UB25 (*Dachangshu*) acupoints, both UB27 (*Xiaochangshu*) acupoints, and both *Yaoyan* extra acupoints in succession, about 40 times each. Then press acupoints UB31-34 (*Baliao*) about 40 times, with the heel of your hand.

Step 7

Press UB37 (*Yinmen*), UB40 (*Weizhong*), UB57 (*Chengshan*), and UB60 (*Kunlun*) acupoints on both legs. Press each pair about 40 times, with your thumbs. Then press pain-relief point G6 on both legs for two minutes.

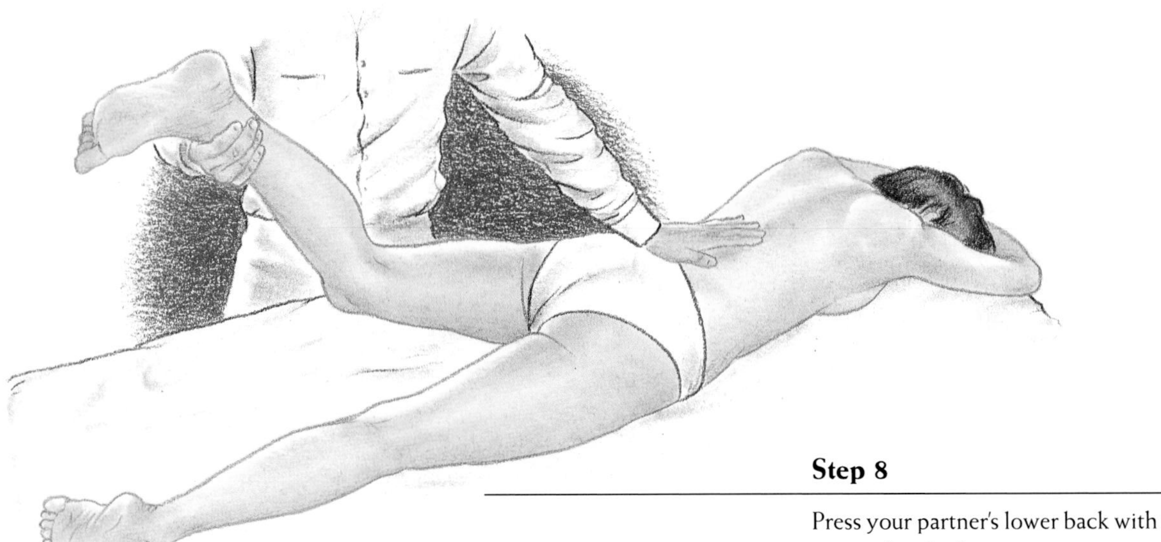

Step 8

Press your partner's lower back with your palm. At the same time, support your partner's right ankle from underneath, and raise the right leg. Lift the leg up and down five to ten times. Repeat on the left leg.

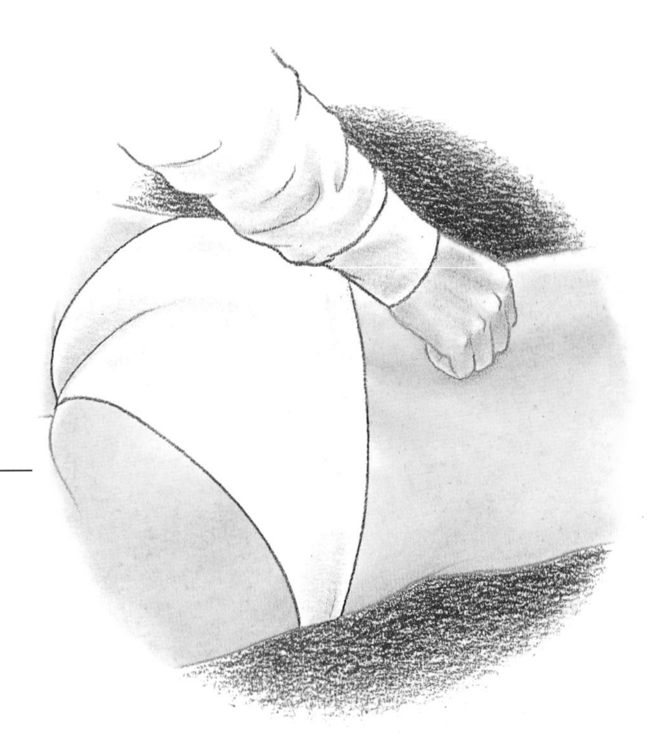

Step 9

Percuss the back about 20 times, with a loosely clenched fist (see also p. 43).

CHRONIC BACK PAIN

This is a long-term condition, and usually has more complicated causes than acute backache (see p. 95). For example, it may be caused by lumbar muscle strain, prolapsed intervertebral disc, rheumatic lumbago, sciatica (see p. 101), or untreated acute lumbar strain.

Chinese medicine indicates that back pain results from injury, or an invasion of Cold and Damp (see p. 9). It may also be the result of a weakness of the Kidneys, neurosis, exhaustion, or very frequent sexual intercourse.

This treatment aims to strengthen the back and the Kidneys. It also improves Qi-blood flow, and expels Cold and Damp. Apply a hot compress to the affected area after treatment for further relief of pain (see p. 30).

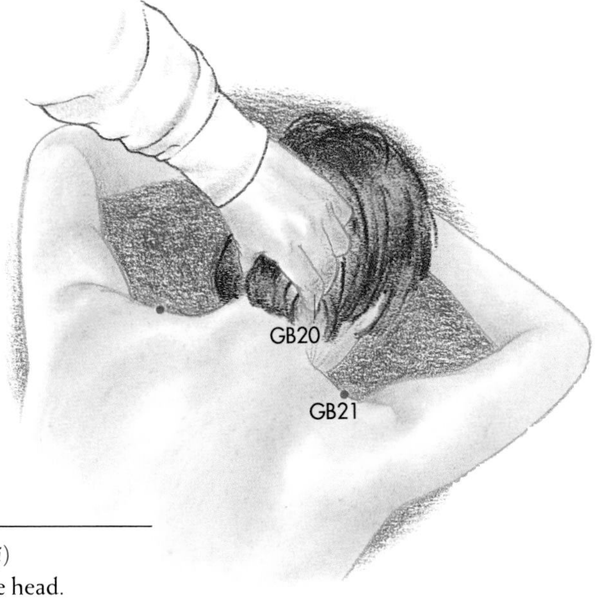

Step 1

Squeeze both GB20 (*Fengchi*) acupoints on the back of the head. Then squeeze both GB21 (*Jianjing*) acupoints 20 to 30 times.

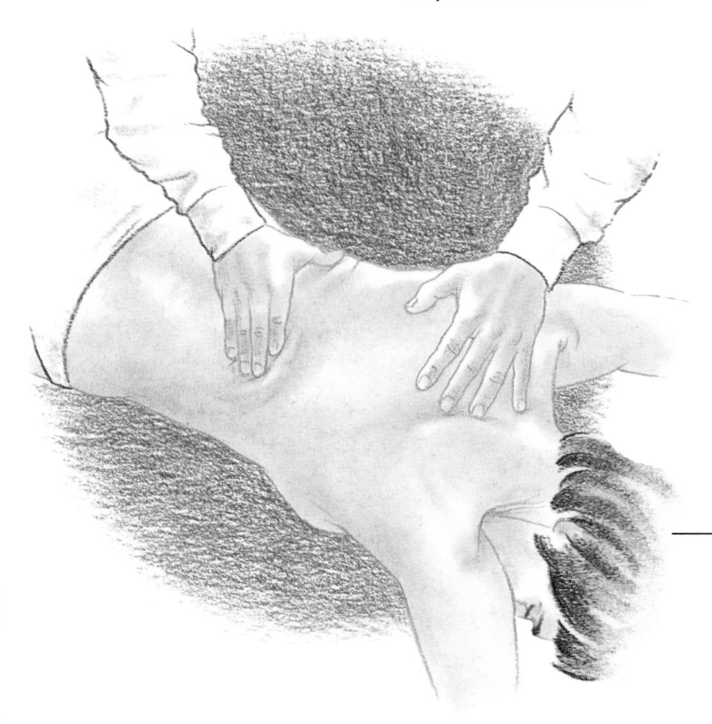

Step 2

Open the Channels in the back region (see pp. 54-6). Take Du4 (*Mingmen*) and UB23 (*Shenshu*) as the major acupoints, and press them a few more times than the others in the sequence, for example, 40 to 50 times each.

Step 3

Push and rub the affected part of the back with one, or both, palms until it feels warm to your partner.

Step 4

Press your partner's lower back with your palm. At the same time, hold your partner's right ankle and raise the right leg. Lift the leg up and down five to ten times. Then repeat on the left leg.

Step 5

Squeeze the muscles down both sides of the back. Then form a pincer shape with your hand, and use it to squeeze the muscles down the back of each leg. Pay particular attention to the muscles in the affected region of the back, and squeeze them for longer.

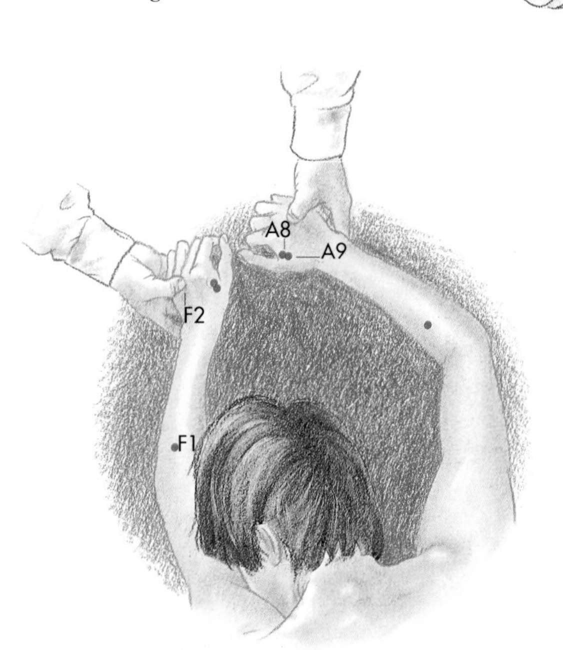

Step 6

Press pain-relief points F1, F2, A8, and A9 on both hands and arms. Use thumb pressure, and press each pair of points for two to three minutes.

Sciatica

To treat back pain caused by sciatica follow Steps 1 to 6 for chronic back pain on pages 99 to 100. Then add the following three steps.

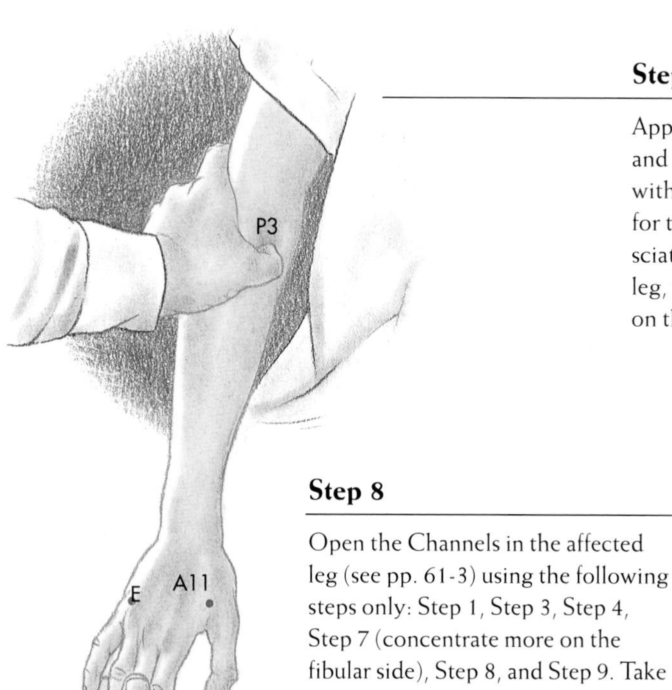

Step 7

Apply pressure to acupoint P3 (*Quze*) and to pain-relief points E and A11 with your thumb. Press each point for two to three minutes. Since sciatica tends to cause pain in one leg, you need only press the points on the affected side.

Step 8

Open the Channels in the affected leg (see pp. 61-3) using the following steps only: Step 1, Step 3, Step 4, Step 7 (concentrate more on the fibular side), Step 8, and Step 9. Take GB31 (*Fengshi*), St34 (*Liangqiu*), GB34 (*Yanglingquan*), GB39 (*Xuanzhong*), and GB40 (*Qiuxu*) as the major acupoints, and press them a few more times than others in the sequence, for example, 40 to 50 times each.

Step 9

Press pain-relief point G6 for two minutes with your thumb.

ACUTE SHOULDER PAIN

According to Chinese medicine, shoulder pain is due to injury of the soft tissue, an invasion of Cold and Damp (see p. 9), or to a hormonal disturbance. It may also be caused by infirmity and weakness, or deficient Qi and blood. Chinese medicine calls this kind of shoulder pain "shoulder pain of the fifties", since middle-aged people often suffer from this problem.

Use this treatment for shoulder pain that has existed for no more than a couple of months. If your partner has experienced pain for more than three months, use the sequence for chronic shoulder pain (see pp. 104-106). Apply very gentle massage strokes to treat acute shoulder pain.

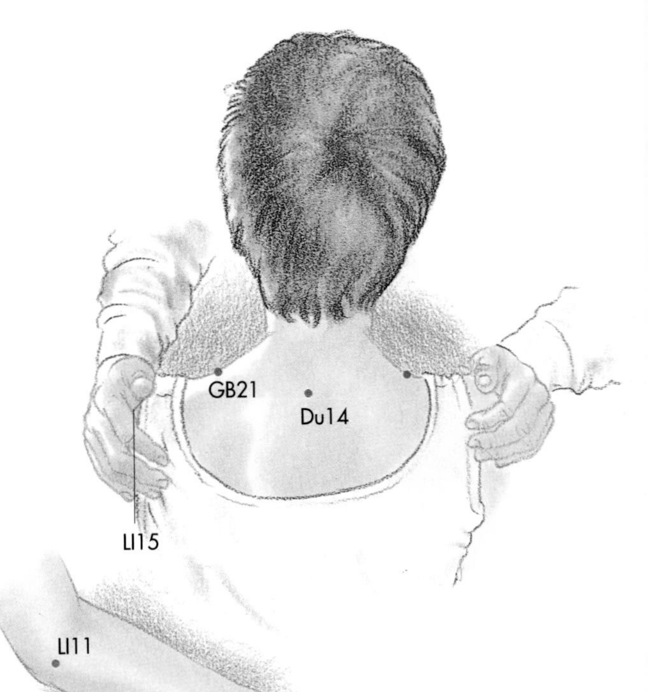

T5

Step 1

Your partner should be seated in a comfortable chair for this massage. Press acupoint Du14 (*Dazhui*) with your thumb. Squeeze acupoint GB21 (*Jianjing*) on both shoulders. Press acupoint LI15 (*Jianyu*) on both shoulders with the heels of your hands. Then press acupoints LI11 (*Quchi*) and T5 (*Waiguan*) on the arm of the affected shoulder. Repeat each manipulation 40 to 50 times.

Step 2

Press and knead the pain-pressure point with the heel of your hand. Ideally, you should use surgical spirits to improve the effect of this massage (see p. 31). Continue massaging the pain-pressure point until it feels warm to your partner.

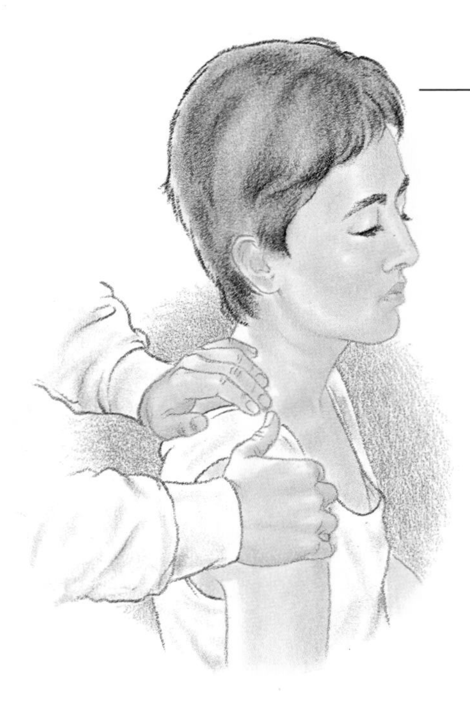

Step 3

Knead and rub the affected shoulder gently with both hands. Use surgical spirits on the shoulder to improve the effect of this massage (see p. 31). Continue kneading and rubbing until the affected shoulder feels warm to your partner.

Step 4

Press pain-relief points B4, A2, A3, and A8 on the arm of the affected side of the body. Press the points one by one with your thumb, for two to three minutes each.

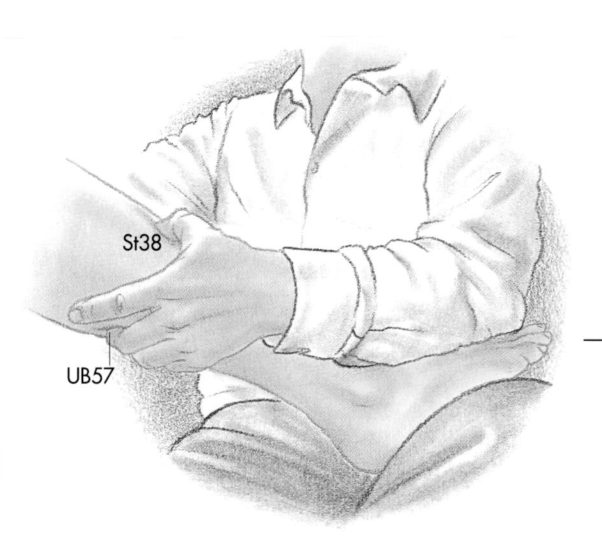

Step 5

Squeeze and press acupoints St38 (*Tiaokou*) and UB57 (*Chengshan*) on the leg of the affected side of the body. Squeeze the two points simultaneously 50 to 100 times.

CHRONIC SHOULDER PAIN

The causes of chronic shoulder pain are the same as acute shoulder pain (see p. 102). Use this pain-relief massage sequence when the pain has persisted for three months or more. If pain exists in only one shoulder, massage the points on the same side of the body as the pain.

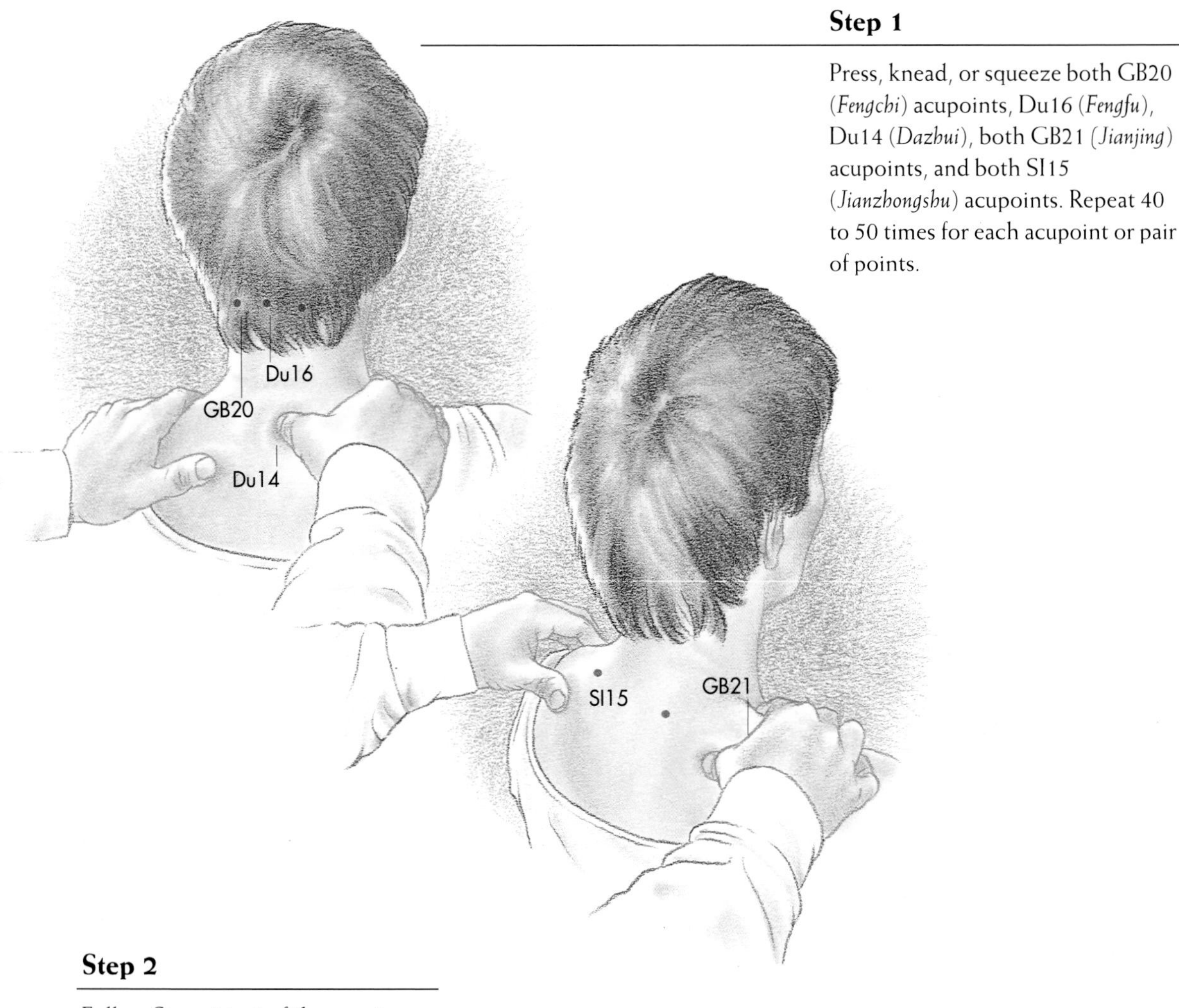

Step 1

Press, knead, or squeeze both GB20 (*Fengchi*) acupoints, Du16 (*Fengfu*), Du14 (*Dazhui*), both GB21 (*Jianjing*) acupoints, and both SI15 (*Jianzhongshu*) acupoints. Repeat 40 to 50 times for each acupoint or pair of points.

Step 2

Follow Steps 1 to 3 of the opening the Channels sequence in the arm region (see pp. 57-8).

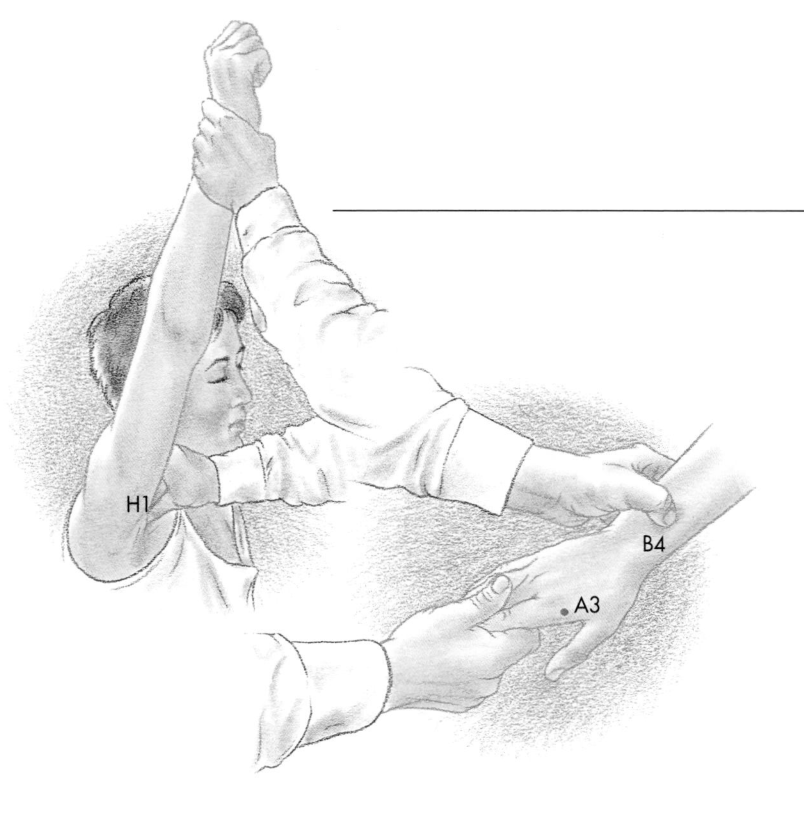

Step 3

Raise the arm of the affected shoulder, and squeeze acupoint H1 (*Jiquan*) 10 times. Then press pain-relief points A3 and B4 on the same arm for two to three minutes each.

Step 4

Squeeze acupoints St38 (*Tiaokou*) and UB57 (*Chengshan*) on the leg of the affected side of the body. Squeeze the two points simultaneously, and repeat 50 to 100 times.

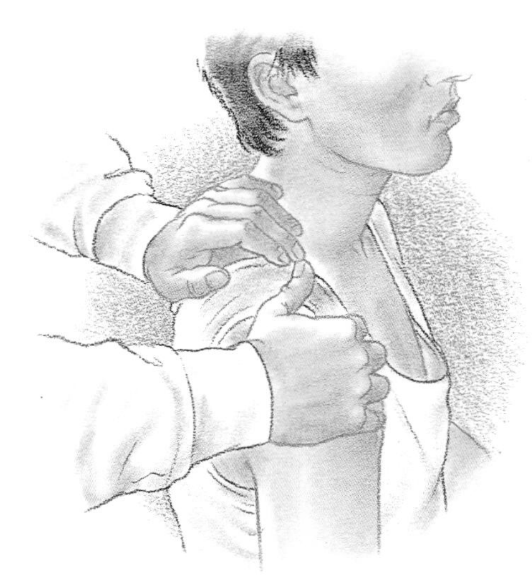

Step 5

Squeeze, knead, and rub the affected shoulder with both palms. Ideally, you should use surgical spirits on the shoulder to improve the effect of this massage (see p. 31). Continue massaging until the shoulder area feels warm to your partner.

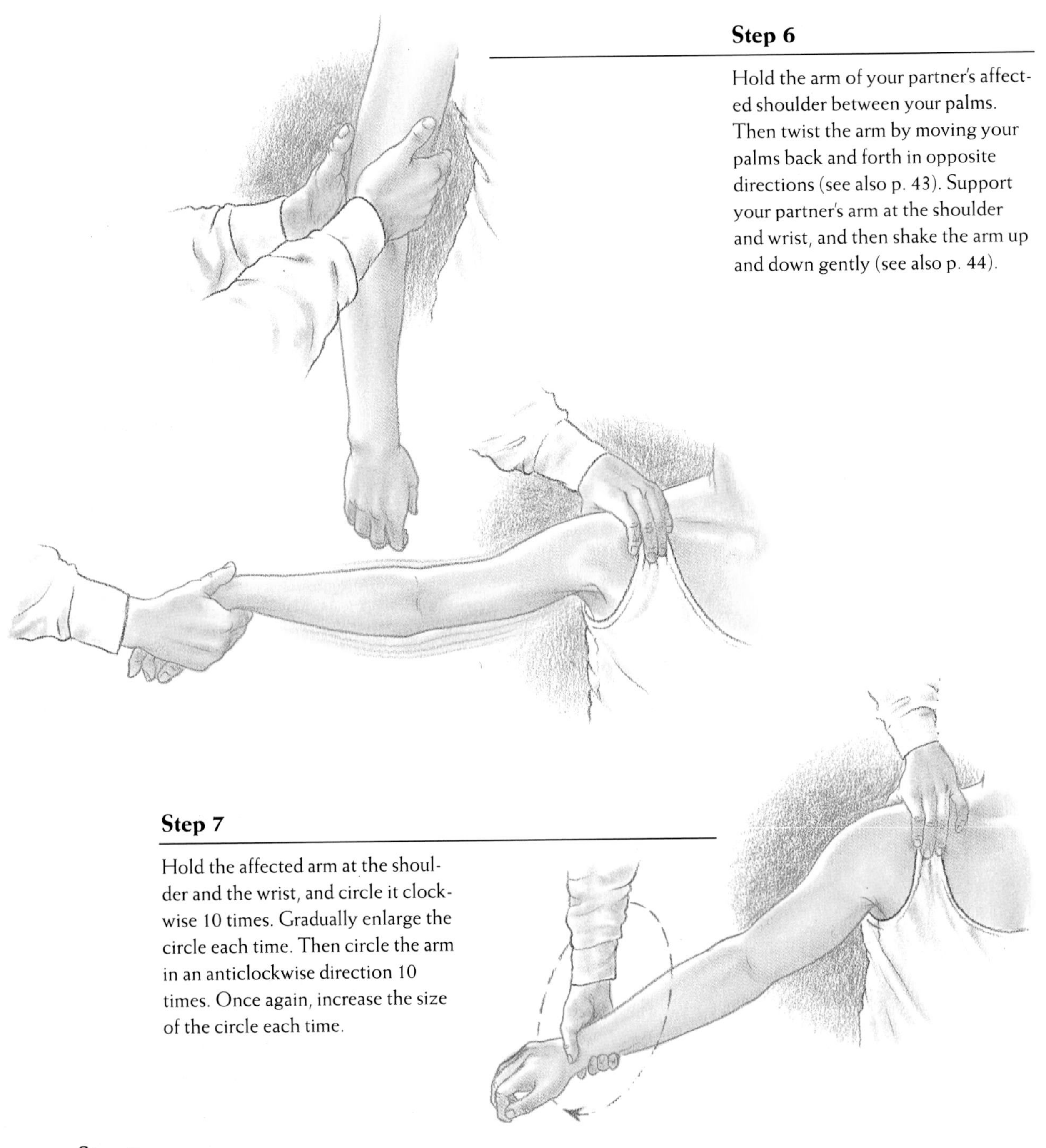

Step 6

Hold the arm of your partner's affected shoulder between your palms. Then twist the arm by moving your palms back and forth in opposite directions (see also p. 43). Support your partner's arm at the shoulder and wrist, and then shake the arm up and down gently (see also p. 44).

Step 7

Hold the affected arm at the shoulder and the wrist, and circle it clockwise 10 times. Gradually enlarge the circle each time. Then circle the arm in an anticlockwise direction 10 times. Once again, increase the size of the circle each time.

Step 8

Squeeze both GB21 (*Jianjing*) acupoints a few times, as in Step 1 (see p. 104).

ELBOW PAIN

The elbow is a shallow hinge joint with a large range of movement. It is supported by overlapping ligaments and tendons. Rapid jerking or small repetitive movements can damage these supporting tissues. The following massage routine is suitable for treating tennis elbow, arthritis, sprains, strains, cramp, and more general aches and pains of the elbow.

CAUTION
REST AN INJURED JOINT FOR 48 HOURS BEFORE TREATMENT, AND SEEK MEDICAL ADVICE BEFORE MASSAGING A DISLOCATED ELBOW.

Step 1

Your partner can be seated for this massage. Gently press the pain-pressure point with your palm. Then knead the whole affected area.

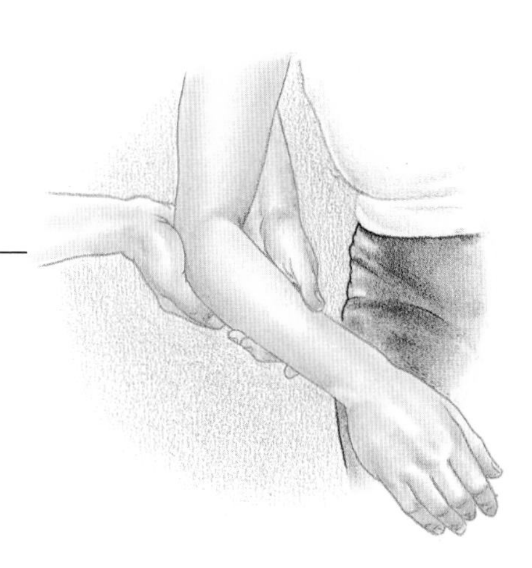

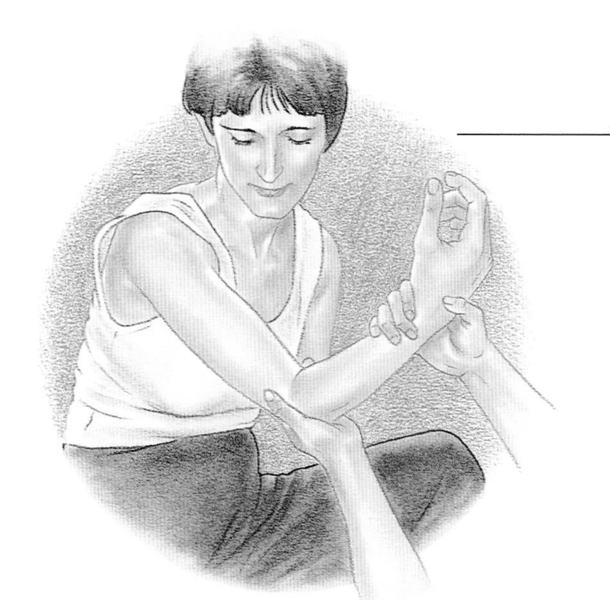

Step 2

Holding the wrist and the elbow, bend and straighten your partner's arm 30 times, stretching it a little each time you straighten it. Then slowly circle the lower arm from the elbow joint (see left). Circle it clockwise 10 times and then anticlockwise 10 times.

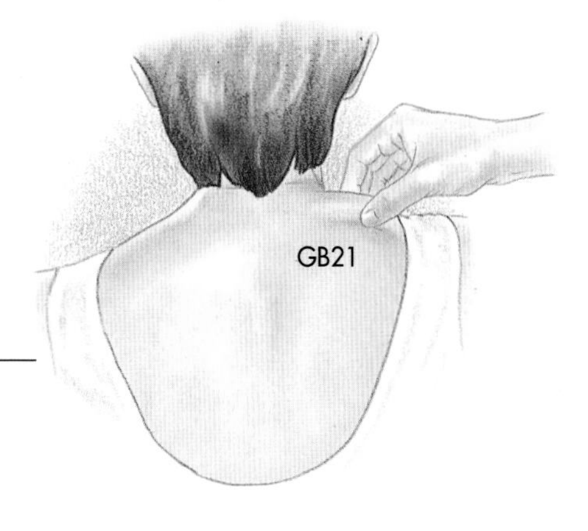

Step 3

Squeeze acupoint GB21 (*Jianjing*), on the affected side of the body 20 times.

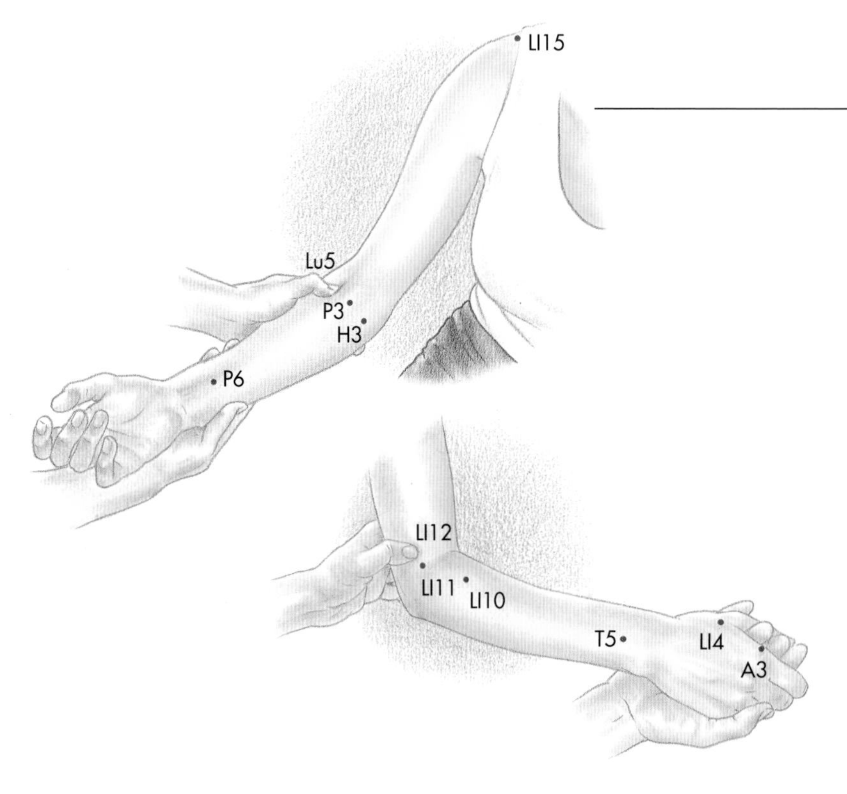

Step 4

Press acupoints LI15 (*Jianyu*), P3 (*Quze*), LI12 (*Zhouliao*), LI11 (*Quchi*), LI10 (*Shousanli*), LI4 (*Hegu*), P6 (*Neiguan*), T5 (*Waiguan*), Lu5 (*Chize*), and H3 (*Shaohai*) on the affected arm. Press the points one by one with your thumb, about 30 times each. Then press pain-relief point A3 on the affected hand for three minutes.

Note: For arthritis replace Step 4 with the sequence for opening the Channels in the back (see pp. 54-6), and in the affected arm (see pp. 57-60). Then press pain-relief point A3 on the affected arm for three minutes.

Step 5

Push and rub the affected elbow with your palms. You can apply surgical spirits (see p. 31) to the elbow to improve the effect of this massage. Continue massaging the elbow until it feels warm to your partner.

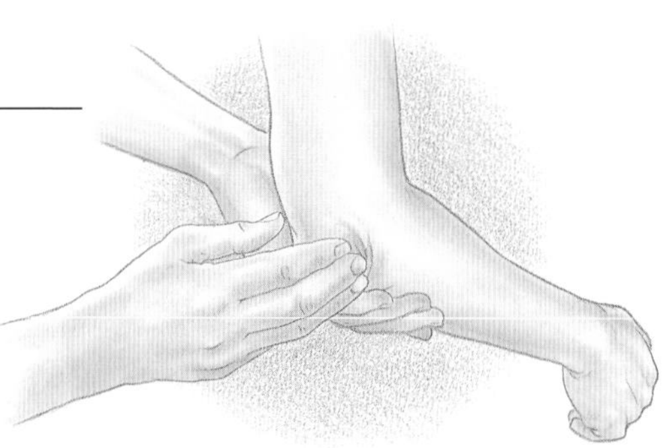

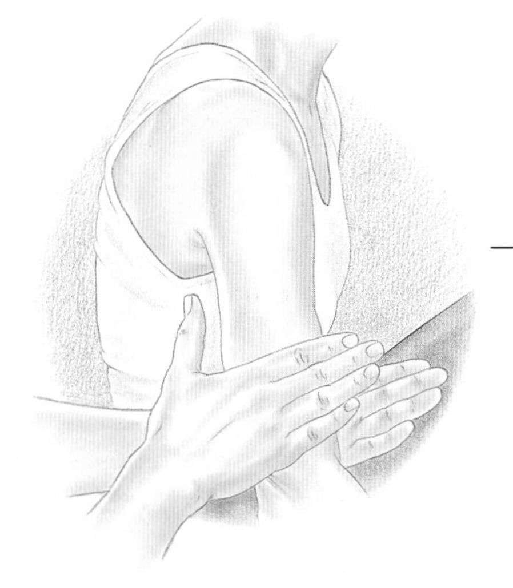

Step 6

Hold the affected elbow between your palms. Twist the arm (see also p. 43) by moving your palms back and forth in opposite directions.

WRIST PAIN

The hand and wrist joints are made up of a complex system of levers and pulleys. They are strong, and allow a wide range of movement. However, the wrist is prone to injury, since you automatically put your hand out to save yourself in a fall. The wrist may also be affected by writer's cramp, a painful spasm caused by repetitive movements such as writing or playing a musical instrument. In addition, arthritis often causes pain and discomfort in the wrist.

CAUTION
REST AN INJURED WRIST FOR 48 HOURS BEFORE TREATING WITH PAIN-RELIEF MASSAGE.

Step 1

Press and squeeze the pain-pressure point gently. Then press and squeeze the whole wrist area.

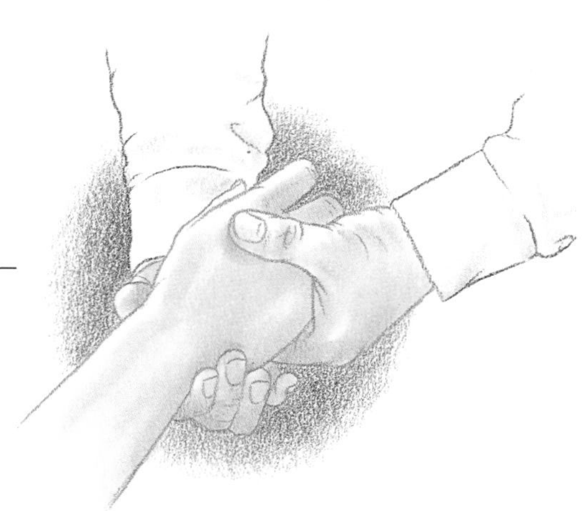

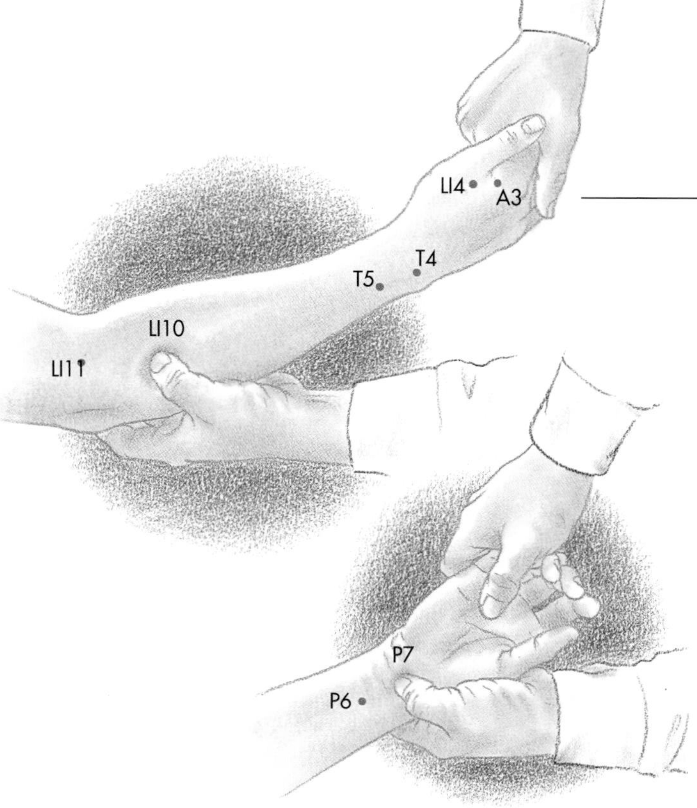

Step 2

With your thumb, press acupoints LI11 (*Quchi*), LI10 (*Shousanli*), T5 (*Waiguan*), P6 (*Neiguan*), T4 (*Yangchi*), P7 (*Daling*), and LI4 (*Hegu*) on the affected arm. Press the points one by one, 30 to 40 times each. Then press pain-relief point A3 for three minutes.

Note: For arthritic wrist pain replace Step 2 with the sequences for opening the Channels in the affected arm (see pp. 57-60), and in the back (see pp. 54-6). Then press point A3 on the affected arm for three minutes.

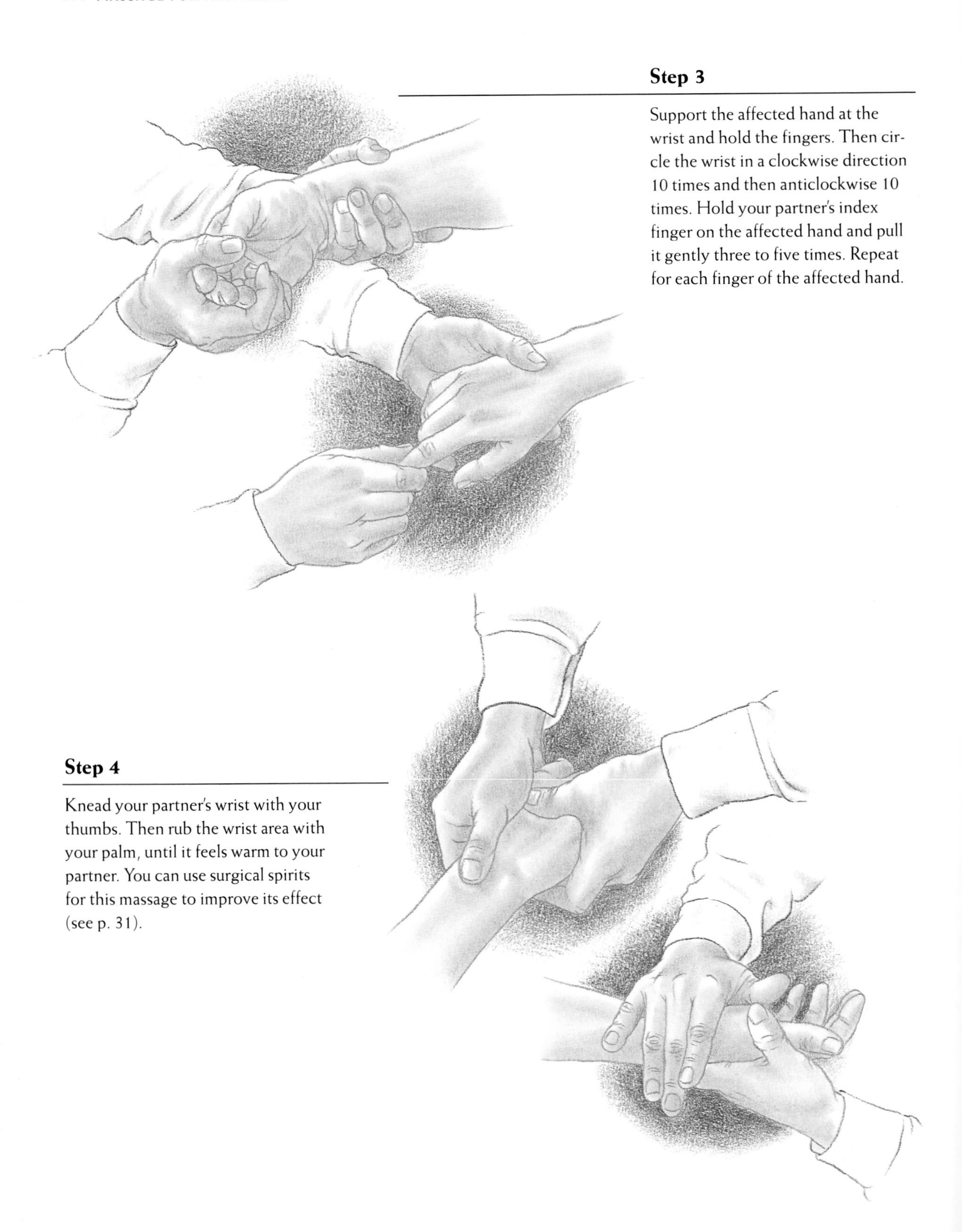

Step 3

Support the affected hand at the wrist and hold the fingers. Then circle the wrist in a clockwise direction 10 times and then anticlockwise 10 times. Hold your partner's index finger on the affected hand and pull it gently three to five times. Repeat for each finger of the affected hand.

Step 4

Knead your partner's wrist with your thumbs. Then rub the wrist area with your palm, until it feels warm to your partner. You can use surgical spirits for this massage to improve its effect (see p. 31).

FINGER PAIN

The fingers are our most useful tool in every-day life, and if misused or overused, they can become strained. Inflammation of the tendon sheath in the hand and arthritis can both cause finger pain. Apply only very gentle massage to treat this problem.

Step 1

With your thumb, press acupoints LI11 (*Quchi*), T5 (*Waiguan*), T4 (*Yangchi*) Lu10 (*Yuji*), P8 (*Laogong*), LI4 (*Hegu*), and SI3 (*Houxi*) on the affected arm. Press the points one by one, 30 to 40 times each.

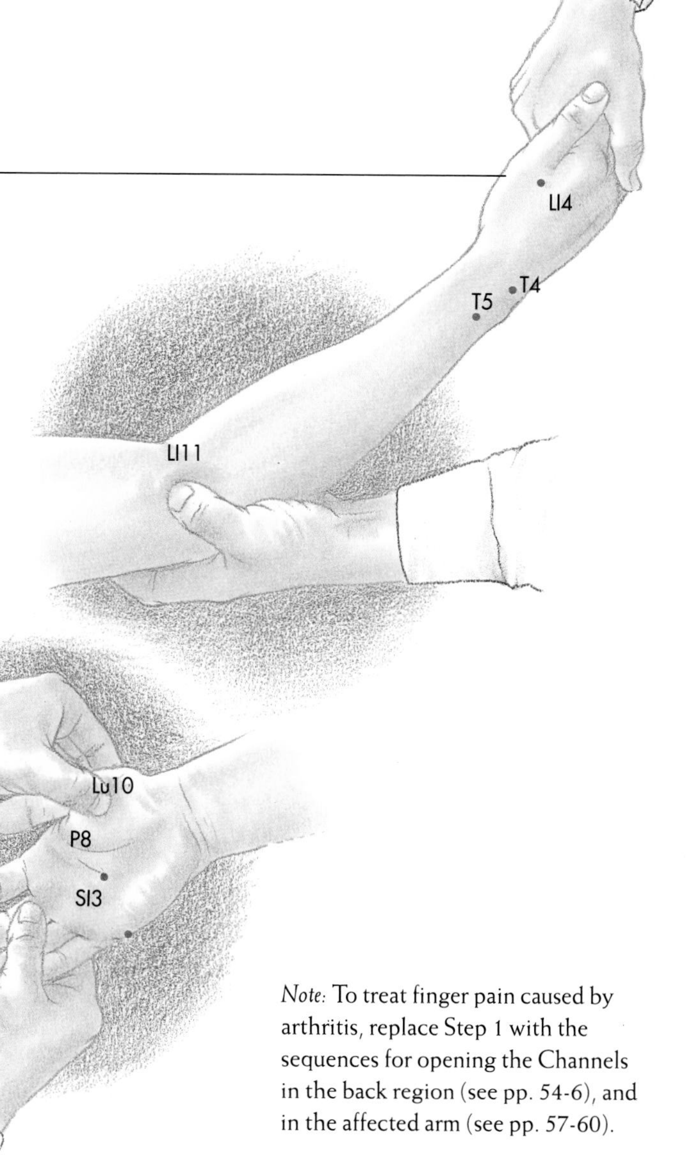

Note: To treat finger pain caused by arthritis, replace Step 1 with the sequences for opening the Channels in the back region (see pp. 54-6), and in the affected arm (see pp. 57-60).

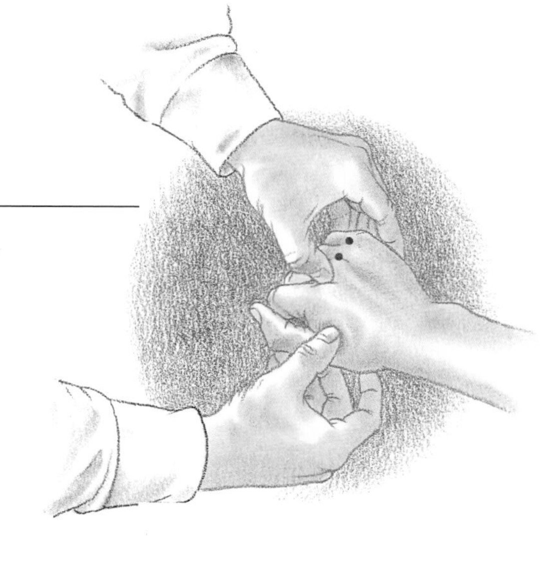

Step 2

With your thumbs, press extra points *Baxie* between the knuckles for two to three minutes each. If you wish, you can press two points at a time.

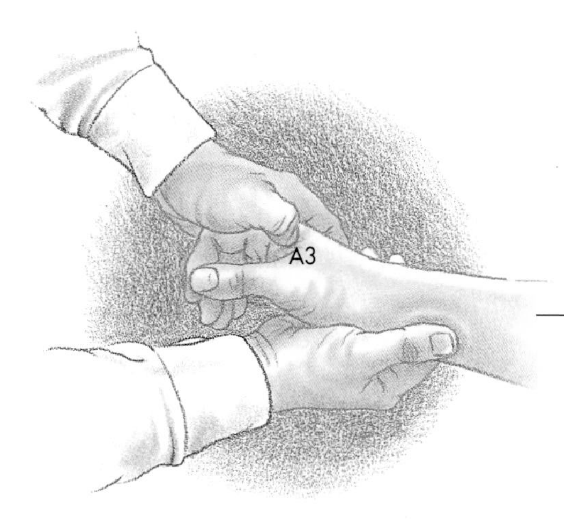

Step 3

Apply thumb pressure to pain-relief point A3 on the affected hand for three minutes.

Step 4

Squeeze the muscles on both sides of the affected arm. Then rub the palm and the back of the hand with your palm. You can apply surgical spirits to the hand to improve this massage (see p. 31). Continue rubbing until the hand feels warm to your partner.

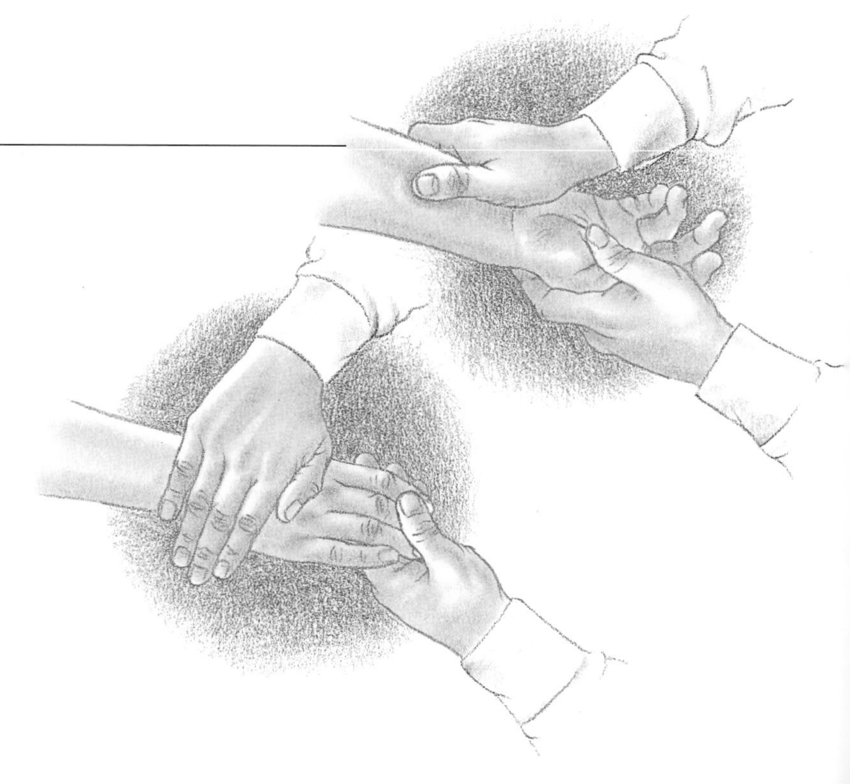

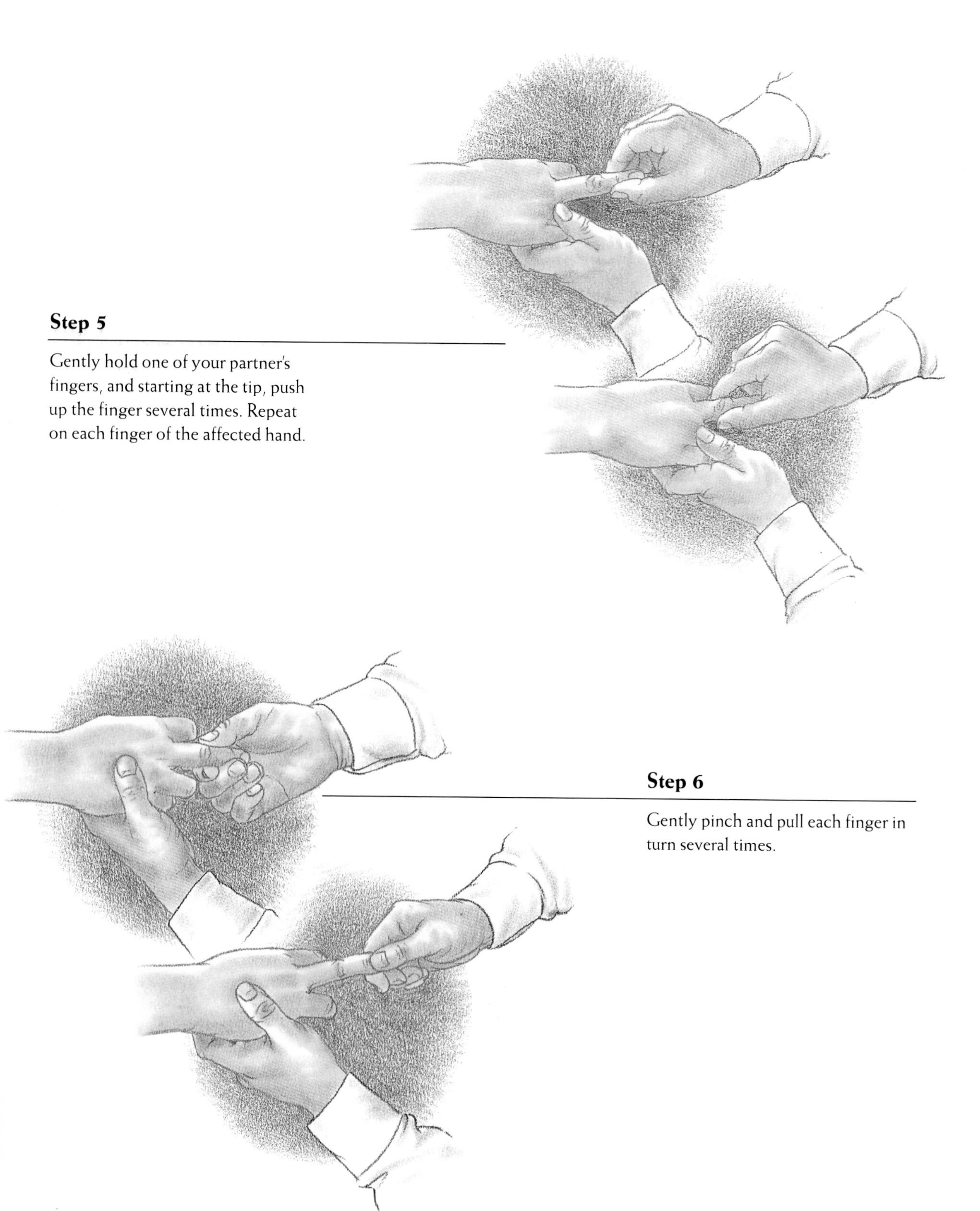

Step 5

Gently hold one of your partner's fingers, and starting at the tip, push up the finger several times. Repeat on each finger of the affected hand.

Step 6

Gently pinch and pull each finger in turn several times.

KNEE PAIN

As weight-bearing joints the knees are subject to physical stress. Use pain-relief massage to treat the knee after injury or strain, and to ease tired and aching knees. Massage can also help to relieve knee pain caused by arthritis.

CAUTION
REST AN INJURED KNEE FOR 48 HOURS BEFORE TREATING WITH PAIN-RELIEF MASSAGE.

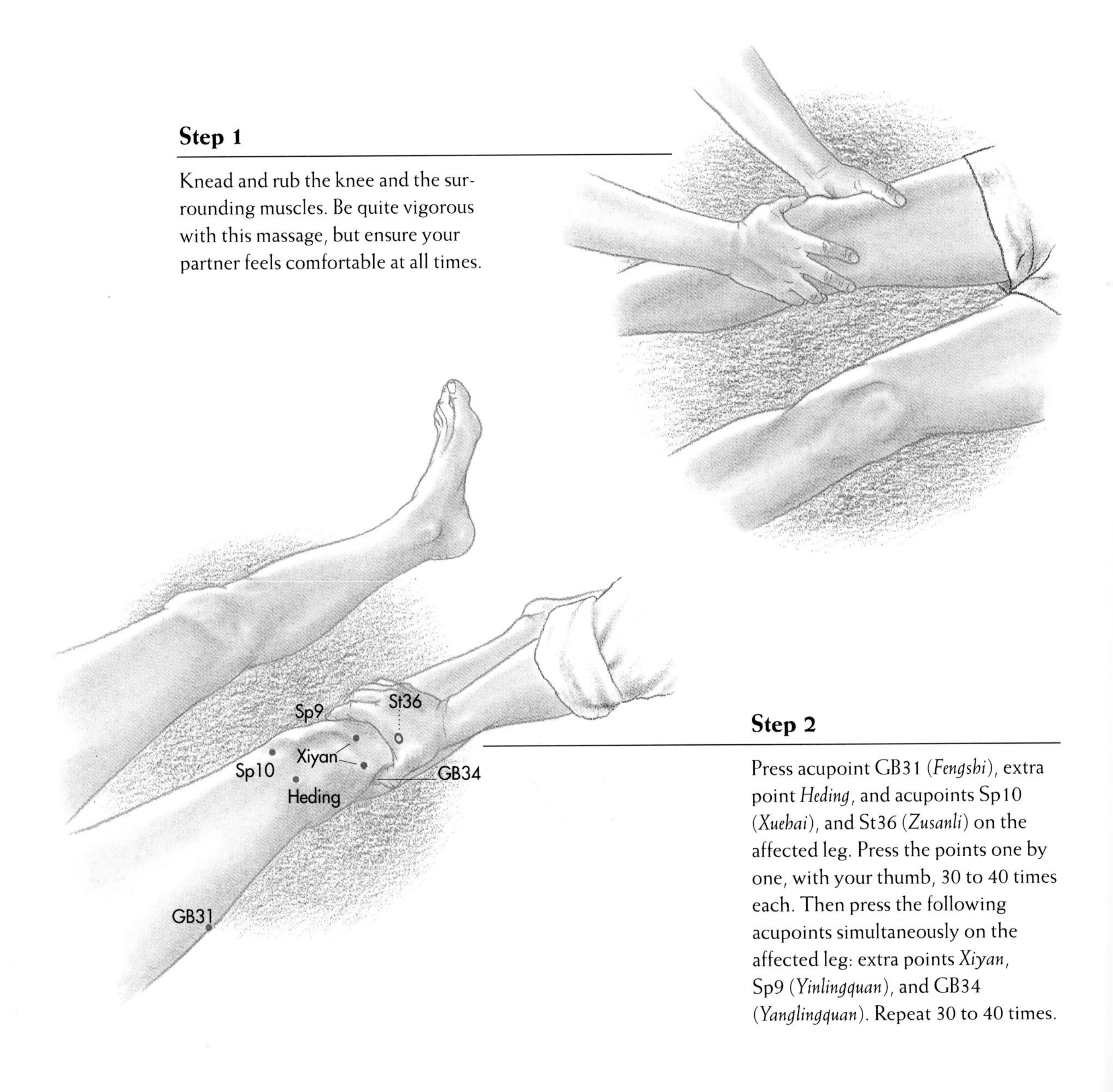

Step 1

Knead and rub the knee and the surrounding muscles. Be quite vigorous with this massage, but ensure your partner feels comfortable at all times.

Step 2

Press acupoint GB31 (*Fengshi*), extra point *Heding*, and acupoints Sp10 (*Xuehai*), and St36 (*Zusanli*) on the affected leg. Press the points one by one, with your thumb, 30 to 40 times each. Then press the following acupoints simultaneously on the affected leg: extra points *Xiyan*, Sp9 (*Yinlingquan*), and GB34 (*Yanglingquan*). Repeat 30 to 40 times.

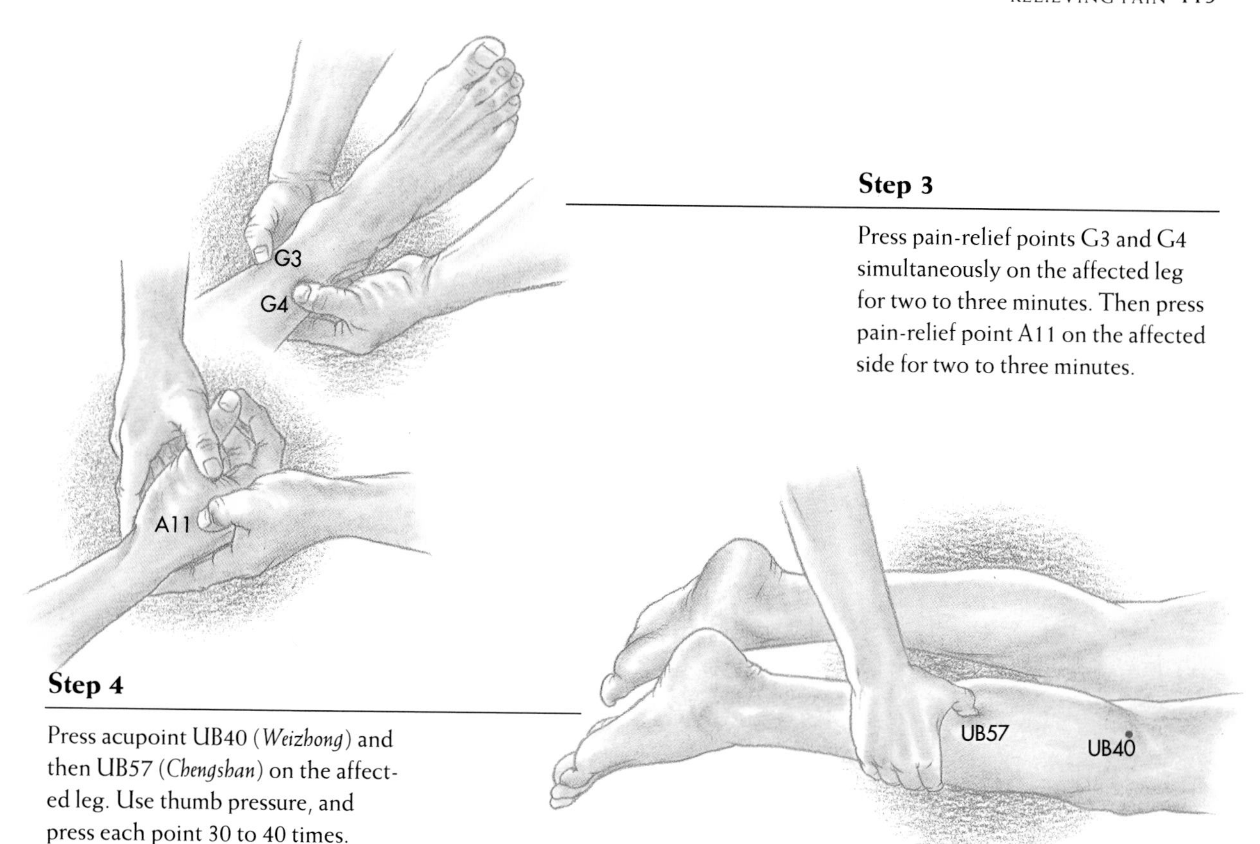

Step 3

Press pain-relief points G3 and G4 simultaneously on the affected leg for two to three minutes. Then press pain-relief point A11 on the affected side for two to three minutes.

Step 4

Press acupoint UB40 (*Weizhong*) and then UB57 (*Chengshan*) on the affected leg. Use thumb pressure, and press each point 30 to 40 times.

Note: If arthritis is the cause of the knee pain, replace Step 2 and Step 4 with the sequence for opening the Channels in the back (see pp. 54-6) and in the affected leg (see pp. 61-3). Take extra points *Heding* and *Xiyan* as the major acupoints, pressing them a few more times than the other points in the sequences, for example, 40 to 50 times each.

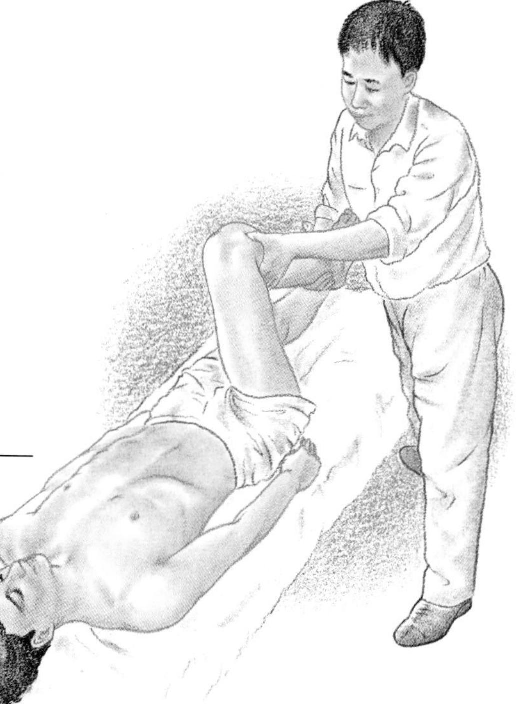

Step 5

With your thumb, press the pain-pressure point of the knee, and hold. At the same time, support the leg at the ankle with your other hand, and bend and straighten the knee joint. Repeat 20 times.

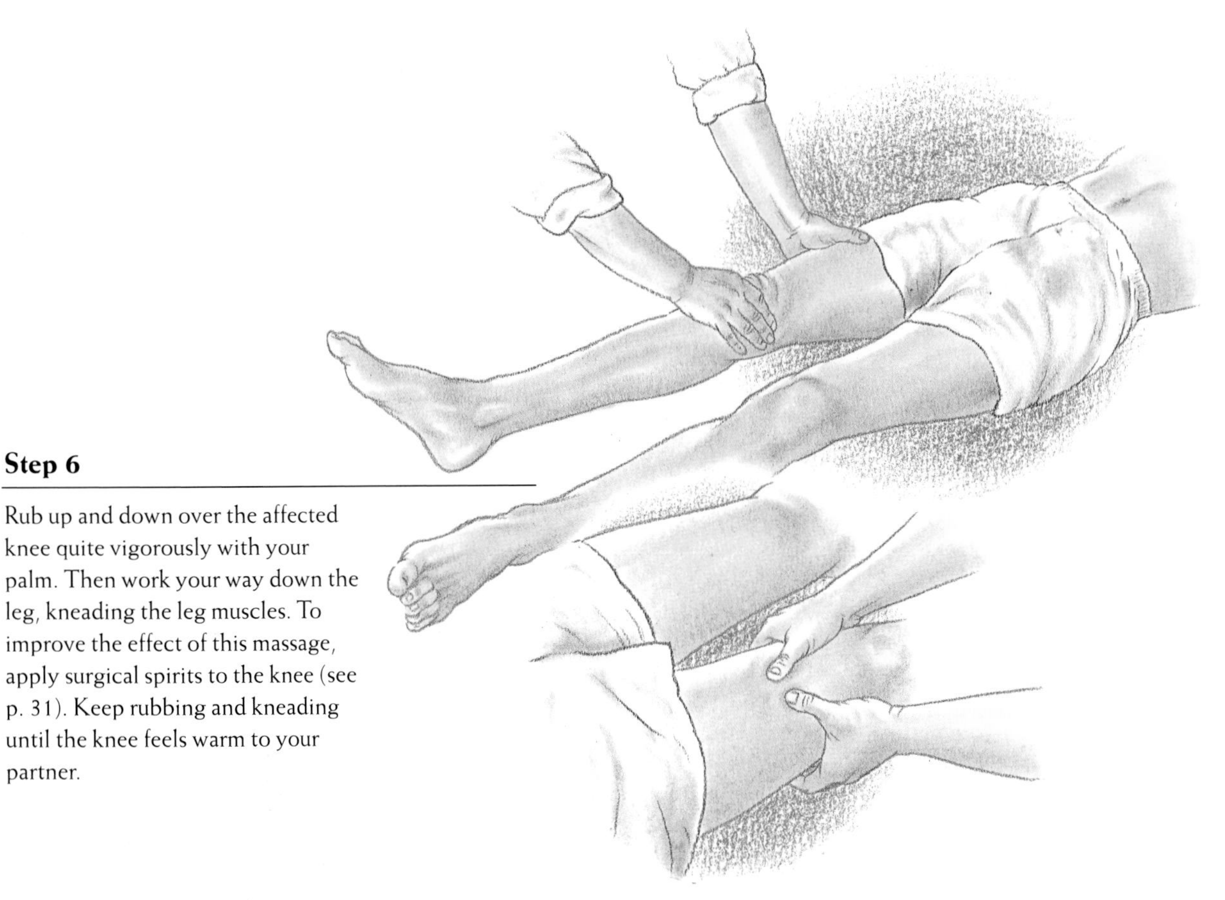

Step 6

Rub up and down over the affected knee quite vigorously with your palm. Then work your way down the leg, kneading the leg muscles. To improve the effect of this massage, apply surgical spirits to the knee (see p. 31). Keep rubbing and kneading until the knee feels warm to your partner.

Step 7

Hold your partner's affected knee between your palms. Twist the knee for about one minute, by moving your palms back and forth in opposite directions (see also p. 43).

ANKLE PAIN

The ankle is a very strong joint with powerful ligaments binding the bones together. It is designed to take your full body weight. However, it is easily twisted, which often causes sprain or ligament damage. A sprained ankle will be swollen and painful. Arthritis may also cause ankle pain.

CAUTION
REST AN INJURED ANKLE FOR 48 HOURS BEFORE TREATING WITH PAIN-RELIEF MASSAGE.

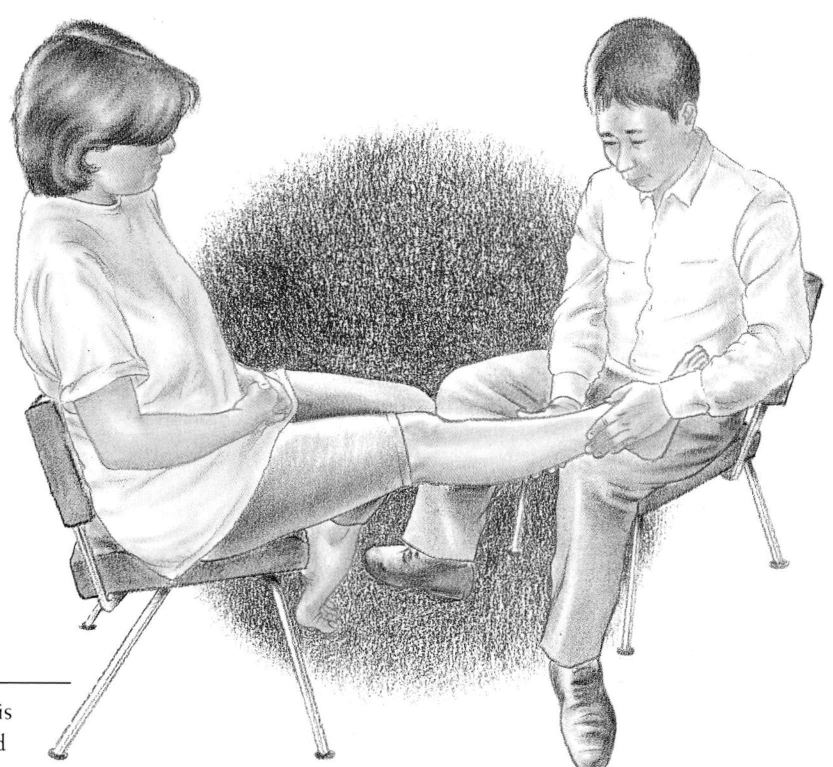

Step 1

Your partner can sit in a chair for this massage sequence, with the affected ankle resting on your knee. Push the ankle with your palms in a centripetal direction, that is, in an upward direction, toward the heart (see p. 29).

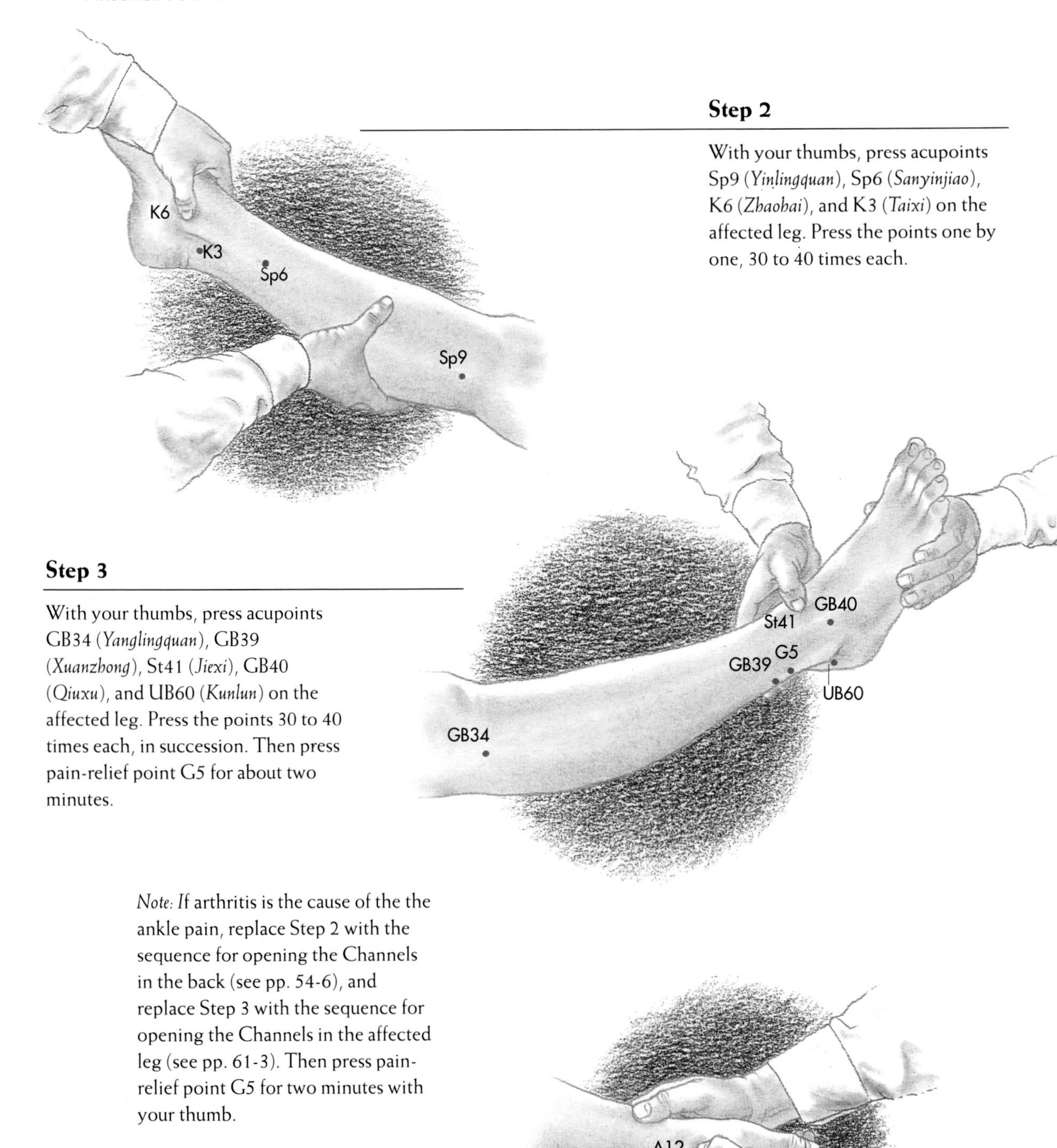

Step 2

With your thumbs, press acupoints Sp9 (*Yinlingquan*), Sp6 (*Sanyinjiao*), K6 (*Zhaohai*), and K3 (*Taixi*) on the affected leg. Press the points one by one, 30 to 40 times each.

Step 3

With your thumbs, press acupoints GB34 (*Yanglingquan*), GB39 (*Xuanzhong*), St41 (*Jiexi*), GB40 (*Qiuxu*), and UB60 (*Kunlun*) on the affected leg. Press the points 30 to 40 times each, in succession. Then press pain-relief point G5 for about two minutes.

Note: If arthritis is the cause of the the ankle pain, replace Step 2 with the sequence for opening the Channels in the back (see pp. 54-6), and replace Step 3 with the sequence for opening the Channels in the affected leg (see pp. 61-3). Then press pain-relief point G5 for two minutes with your thumb.

Step 4

Press pain-relief point A12 on the affected side of the body for three minutes with your thumb.

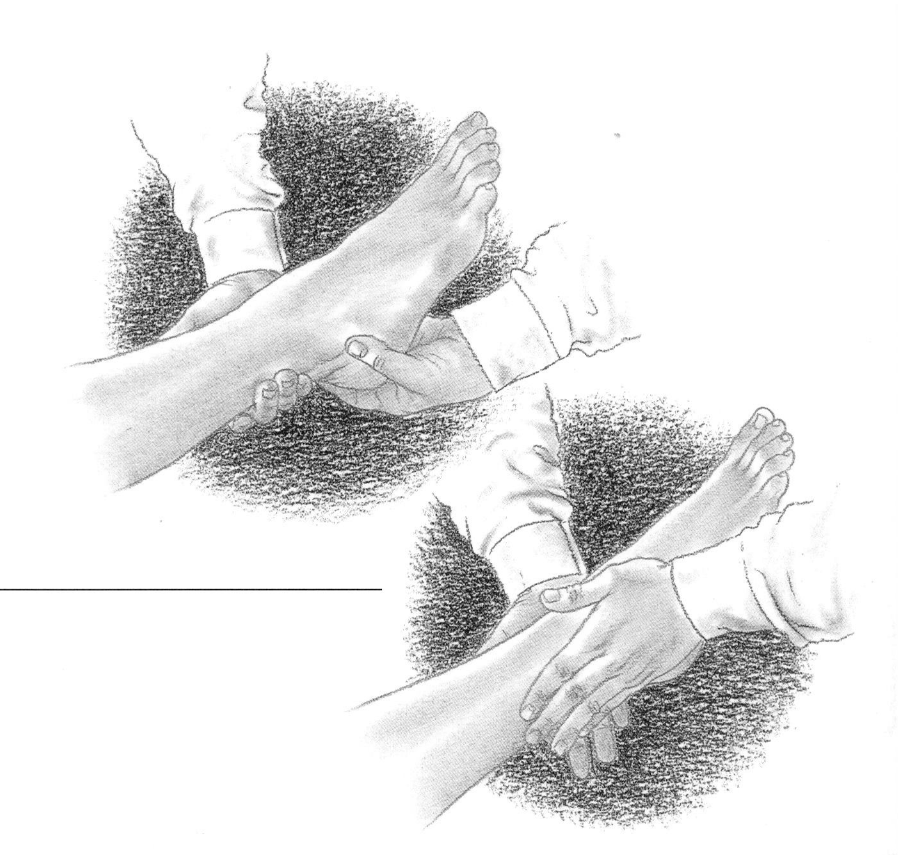

Step 5

Press the pain-pressure point and then push and knead the area until it feels warm to your partner. Ideally, you should use surgical spirits for this step to improve the effect of the massage (see p. 31).

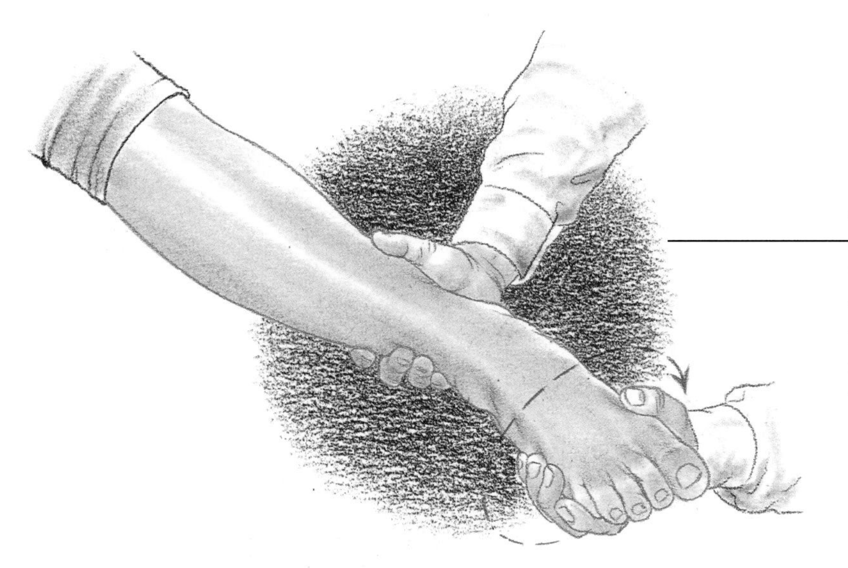

Step 6

Gently circle the ankle joint 10 times in a clockwise direction. Then repeat in an anticlockwise direction. Then flex and straighten the ankle 10 times.

HEEL PAIN

Heel pain is a common complaint for middle-aged and older people. It is often caused by atrophy of the fat pad under the heel. Overweight people may also be prone to this problem.

Pain-relief massage can help. Your partner should also soak the affected foot in hot water for 20 minutes every evening to improve the effect of the treatment.

Step 1

Your partner should be lying on his or her back for this massage. Hold the ankle and raise the leg slightly. Then press and squeeze the pain-pressure point.

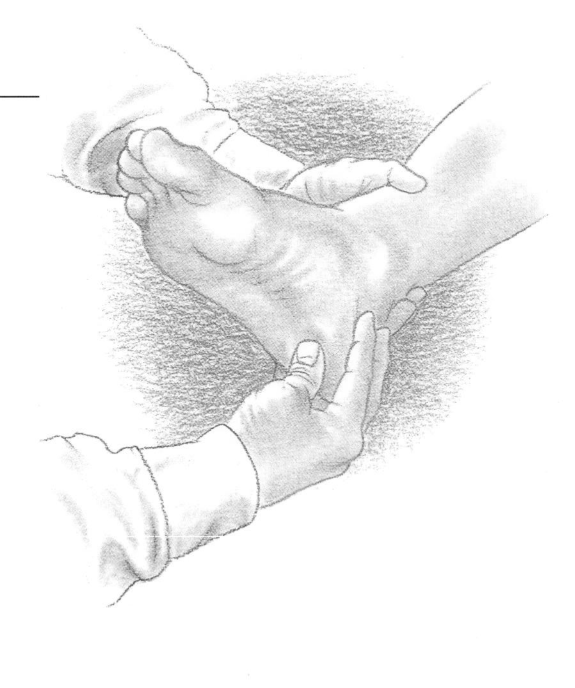

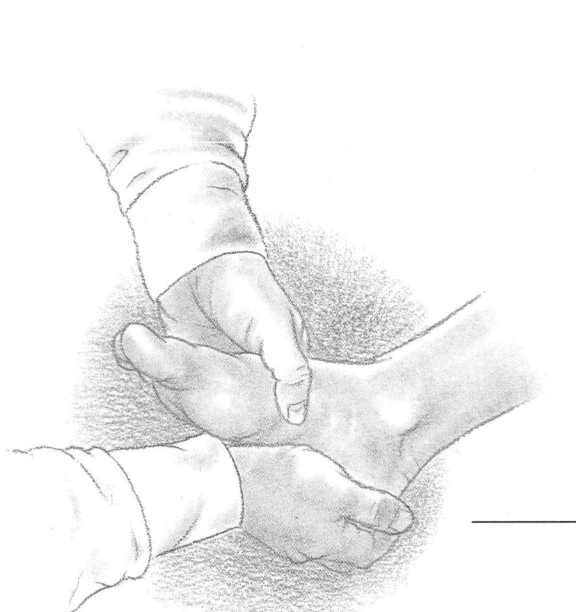

Step 2

With your palm, slowly push down the sole of the foot from the toes to the heel. Apply some pressure, and repeat 30 times.

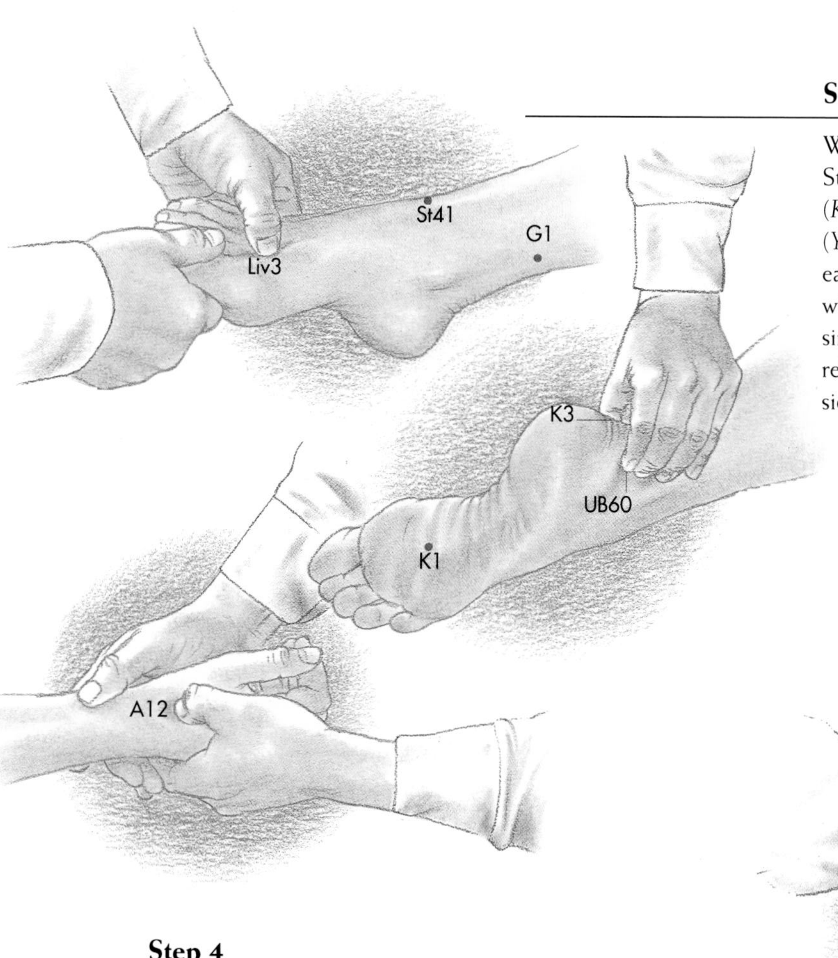

Step 3

With your thumb, press acupoints St41 (*Jiexi*), K3 (*Taixi*), UB60 (*Kunlun*), Liv3 (*Taichong*), and K1 (*Yongquan*) on the affected leg. Press each point 30 to 40 times. If you wish, you can press K3 and UB60 simultaneously. Then press pain-relief points G1 and A12 in succession, for two minutes each.

Step 4

Squeeze the whole heel area 20 times.

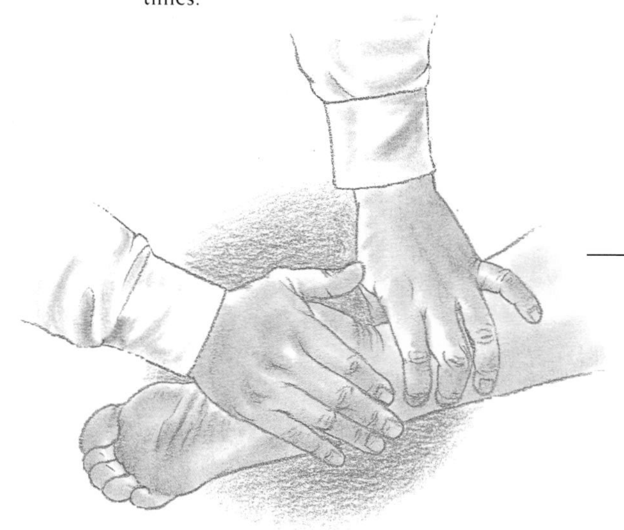

Step 5

With your palm, rub up and down over the sole and heel of the foot. Repeat about 50 times.

APPENDIX

THE CHANNELS

EACH CHANNEL FOLLOWS A SPECIFIC COURSE THROUGH THE BODY. THE ILLUSTRATIONS SHOW THE SUPERFICIAL COURSE OF EACH CHANNEL ON THE SURFACE OF THE BODY, AND THE WRITTEN DESCRIPTIONS SUPPLEMENT THIS WITH DETAILS ON THEIR INTERNAL COURSE. THE TYPICAL SYMPTOMS OF CHANNEL DISTURBANCE (SEE PP. 8-13) ARE ALSO GIVEN HERE.

The Lung Channel of Hand-Taiyin

This Channel starts at the Middle Warmer (see p. 9), and descends to meet its paired Yang organ, the Large Intestine, and then the Stomach and the Lungs. It then passes the armpit, and surfaces in front of the shoulder. The Channel travels along the radial border of the front of the arm, and ends at the corner of the thumbnail. Eleven acupoints are located on the Lung Channel.

Symptoms of disease in the Channel

Thirst, cough, spitting or coughing up blood, tightness and pressure in the chest, difficulty in breathing, feeling ill at ease, frequent urination and dark urine, pain in the collarbone area, shoulder, and upper back, feverish sensation of the palm, and local symptoms along the course of the Channel.

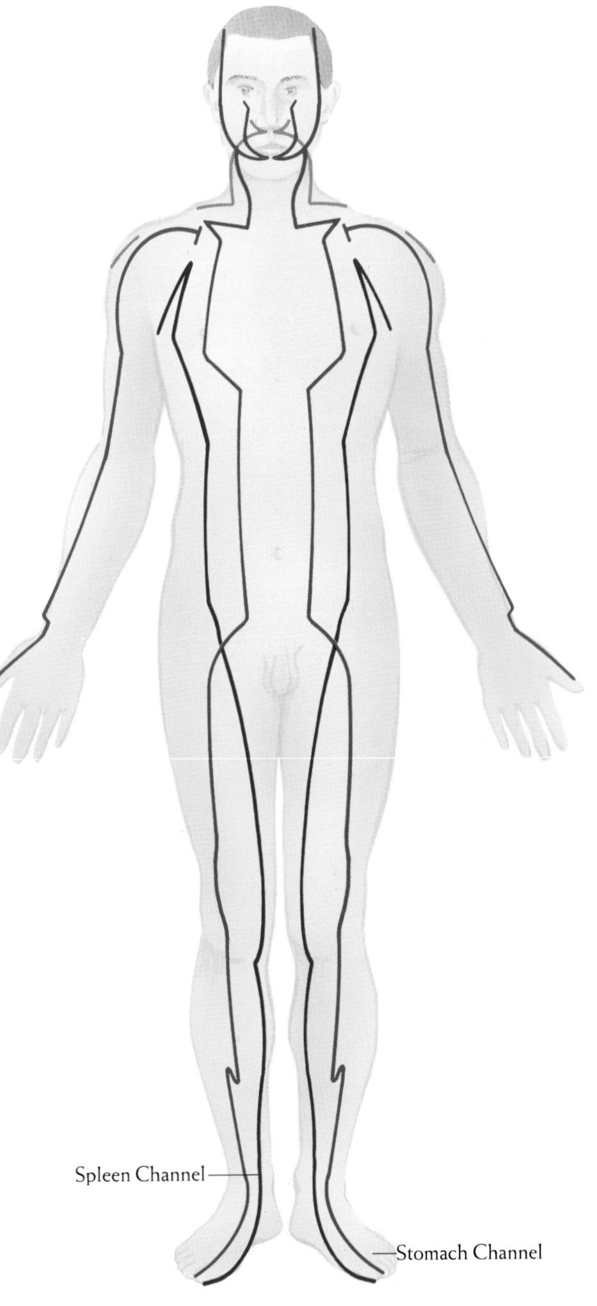

The Large Intestine Channel of Hand-Yangming

The Large Intestine Channel starts at the tip of the index finger. It passes through the back of the hand, via the radial border of the back of the arm, and up to the shoulder and the 7th cervical vertebra. The Channel then curves through the depression behind the collarbone and descends internally to connect with the Lung, and its own organ, the Large Intestine. The Channel travels upward through the neck and cheek from the shoulder, and ends by the wing of the nose. The Lung Channel has 20 acupoints along its course.

Symptoms of disease in the Channel:

Diarrhoea, constipation, toothache, dryness in the mouth, nosebleeds, sore throat, swelling in the neck, and other local symptoms along the course of the Channel.

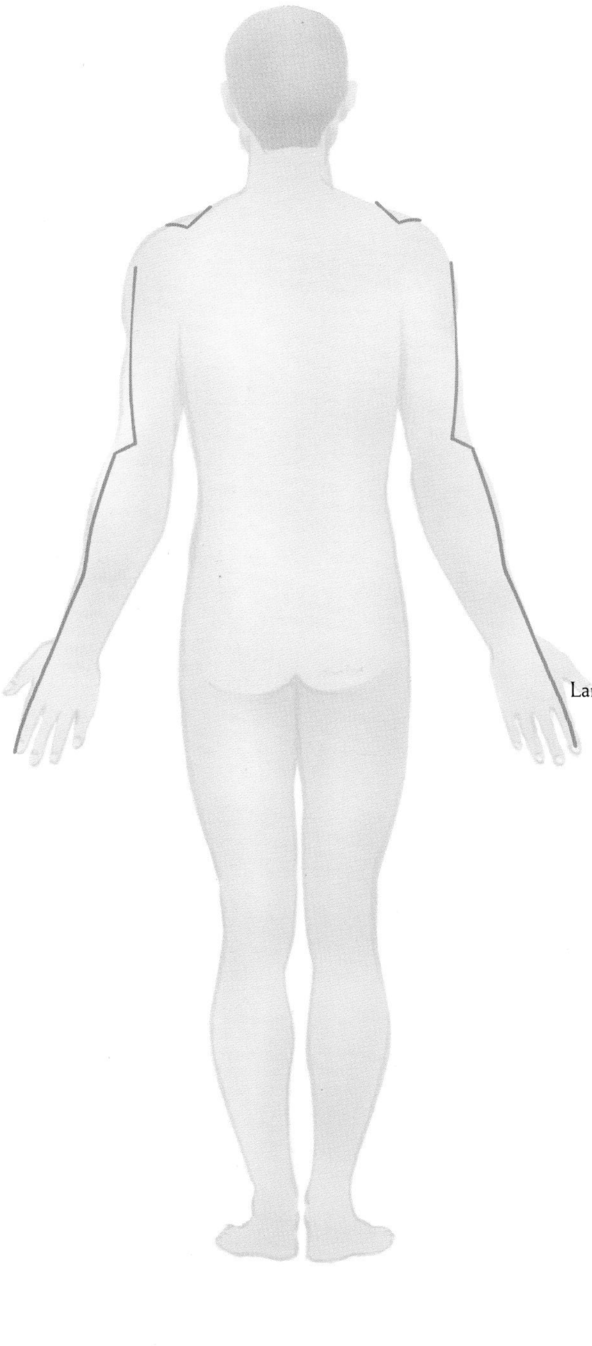

The Stomach Channel of Foot-Yangming

From its starting point by the wing of the nose, the Stomach Channel extends in a "U" shape, with one end at the bridge of the nose, and the other extending along the cheek and up the forehead. From the jaw, the Channel moves alongside the throat to the collarbone region, where it divides. One branch descends internally to meet the Stomach and the Spleen. The other branch descends over the abdomen to the pubic area, where at acupoint St30 (*Qichong*) it meets a second internal branch. It then runs down the front of the leg, and ends at the tip of the second toe. There are 45 acupoints along this Channel.

Symptoms of disease in the Channel:
Stomachache, flatulence, vomiting, thirst, sore throat, nosebleeds, palpitations, swelling in the neck, fever, and local pain along the course of the Channel.

Large Intestine Channel

The Spleen Channel of Foot-Taiyin

The Spleen Channel begins at the tip of the big toe, and climbs up the inside of the leg. It enters the abdominal cavity and meets with the Spleen and the Stomach, where it divides. The internal branch goes to the Heart, while the main branch continues up through the abdomen to the tongue. There are 21 acupoints on the Spleen Channel.

Symptoms of disease in the Channel
Stomachache, indigestion, vomiting, abdominal distension and bloating, loss of appetite, pain and stiffness of the tongue, jaundice, and a feeling of tiredness and heaviness in the body.

The Heart Channel of Hand-Shaoyin

This Channel starts from its own organ the Heart, and descends internally to link with the Small Intestine, its related organ. One branch goes upward from the Heart, and forms a net around the eye. Another branch passes through the Lung, and surfaces at the armpit. It then runs down the ulnar side of the arm to the tip of the little finger. Nine acupoints are located along the Heart Channel.

Symptoms of disease in the Channel

Cardiac pain, chest pain, thirst, dry throat, yellow discolouration of the eyes, feverish sensation in the palm, and local symptoms along the course of the Channel.

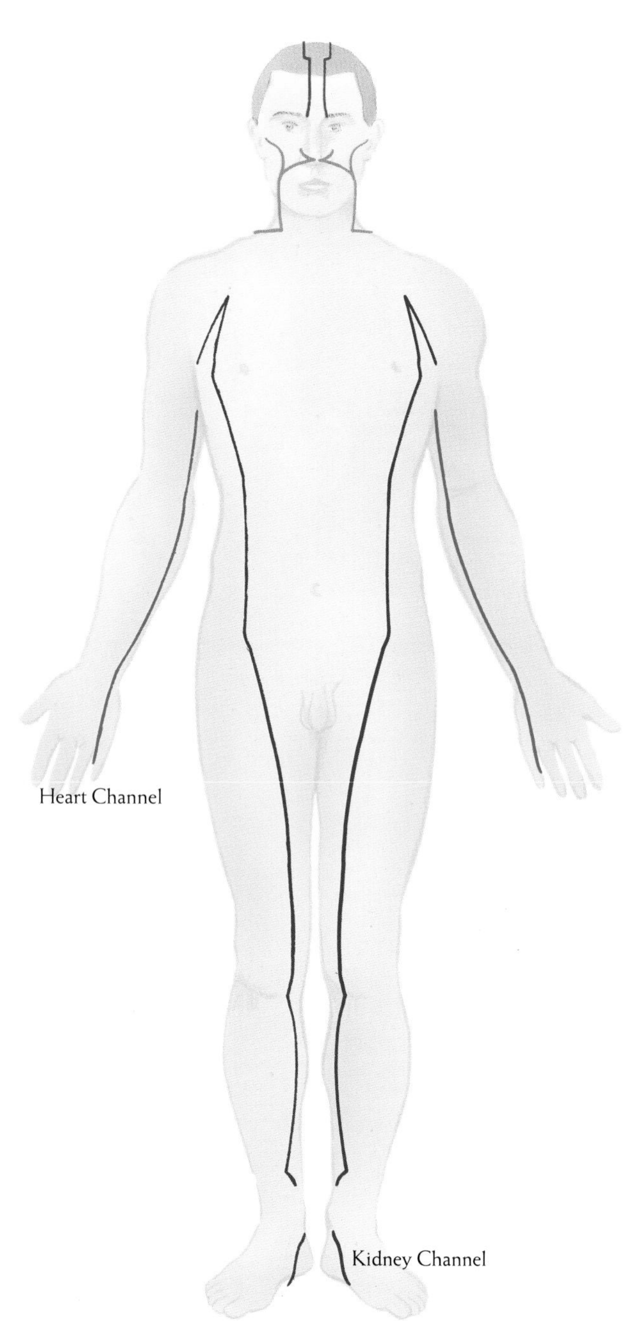

The Small Intestine Channel of Hand-Taiyang

This Channel starts at the tip of the little finger, and runs along the ulnar border of the back of the arm to the shoulder and the 7th cervical vertebra. It divides in the collarbone region. An internal branch descends to meet the Heart, Stomach, and finally its own organ, the Small Intestine. From the collarbone, the other branch runs up the side of the neck to the cheek, where it divides – one branch goes to the outer corner of the eye and then to the ear. The other branch extends to touch the inner corner of the eye. There are 19 acupoints along the Small Intestine Channel.

Symptoms of disease in the Channel

Impairment of hearing, yellow discolouration of the eyes, swelling of the jaws and cheeks, and other local symptoms along its pathway, such as pain in the jaw, neck, shoulder, elbow, and arm.

The Urinary Bladder Channel of Foot-Taiyang

Starting at the inner corner of the eye, the Urinary Bladder Channel passes over the forehead up to the top of the head, at which point it branches to touch the ear. The second branch goes straight down to the occipital bone, where it enters the skull, and connects with the brain. After passing the nape, the Channel descends parallel to the spine to the lumbar region. At the acupoint UB23 (*Shenshu*), it penetrates deeper to meet the Urinary Bladder and the Kidney. A third branch descends from the lumbar region to the back of the knee. The last branch diverges from the main Channel at the nape, and also runs parallel to the spine (the second line from the spine). It passes down the back of the leg, and joins the third branch at the back of the knee. It finishes at the tip of the little toe. There are 67 acupoints along this Channel.

Symptoms of disease in the Channel

Fever, eye problems including yellowing of the eyes and watery eyes, nosebleeds, headache, stiffness and pain in the neck, back, and legs, frequent urination, and difficult or painful urination.

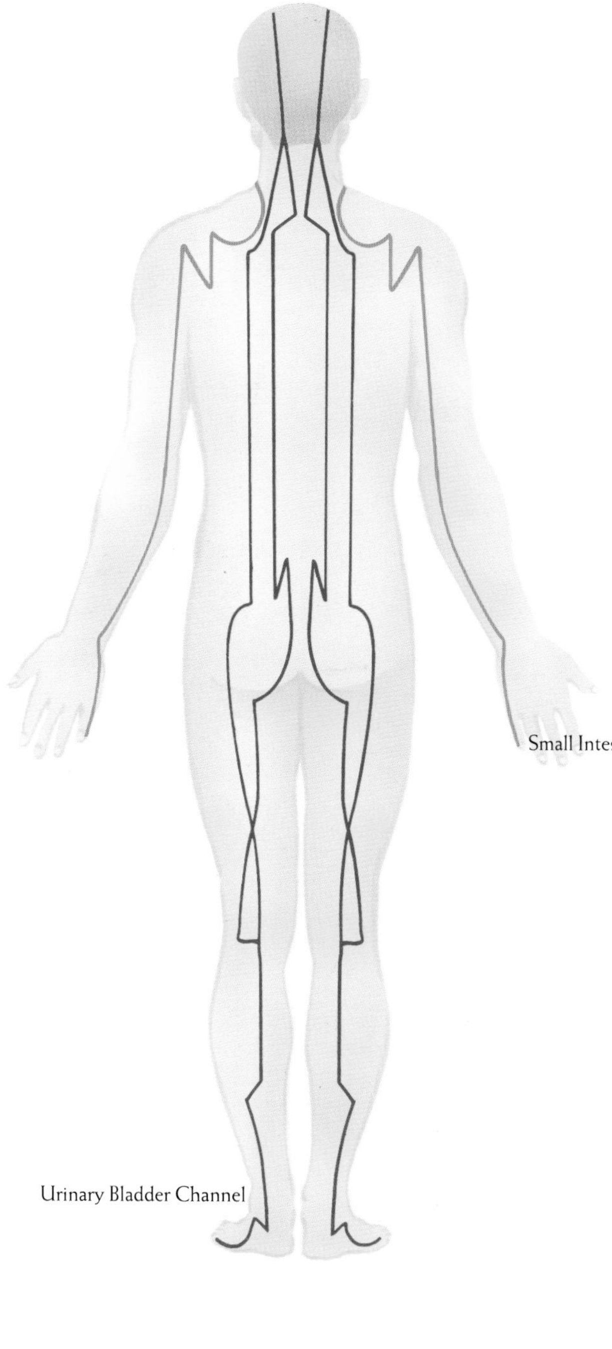

Small Intestine Channel

The Kidney Channel of Foot-Shaoyin

This Channel starts at the little toe, and passes along the sole of the foot before proceeding up the inside of the leg to the top of the inner thigh. From here it follows a deeper, internal path, which takes it to the Kidney and the Urinary Bladder. One branch starts at the Kidney and passes through the Liver, Lungs, and throat up to the tongue. The other branch starts at the Lung and meets the Heart. There are 27 acupoints on the Kidney Channel.

Symptoms of disease in the Channel

Dry tongue, sore throat, spitting or coughing up blood, difficulty in breathing, diarrhoea, constipation, oedema, and local symptoms along the path of the Channel.

Urinary Bladder Channel

The Pericardium Channel of Hand-Jueyin

The Pericardium Channel starts in the chest and meets with the Pericardium. It then crosses the diaphragm, and passes through the Triple Warmer region (see p. 9). Its main branch emerges from the abdomen just outside the nipple, and flows down the arm to end at the tip of the middle finger. Nine acupoints are located along the Pericardium Channel.

Symptoms of disease in the Channel

Cardiac pain, palpitations, fullness and tightness in the chest, flushed complexion, yellow discolouration of the eyes, feeling ill at ease, mental disorder, and local symptoms along the course of the Channel.

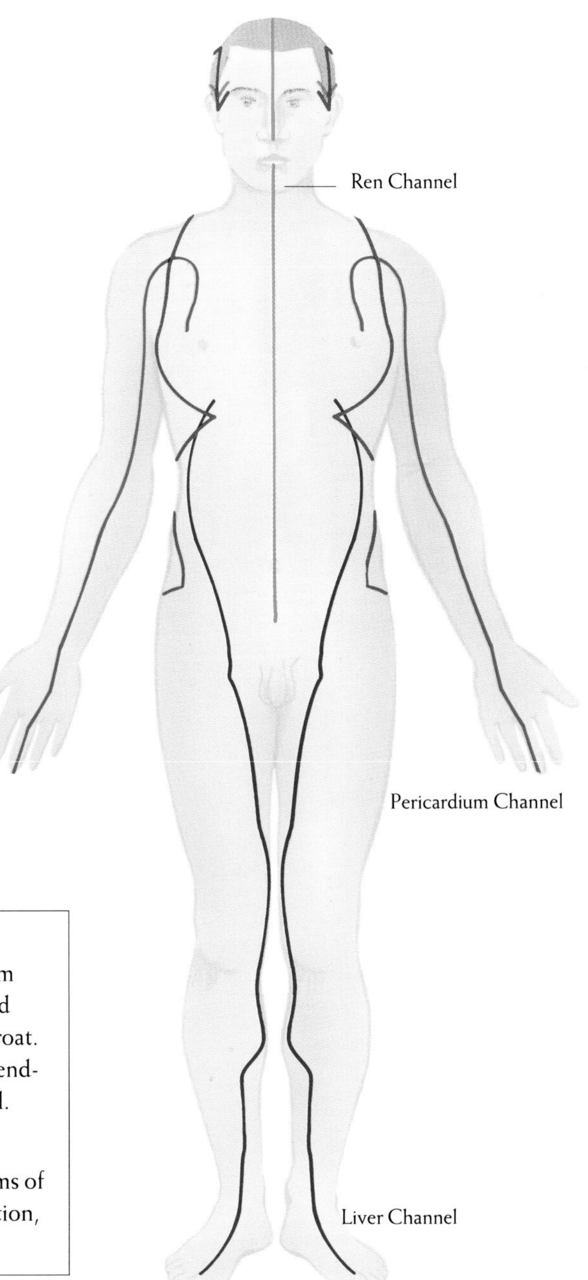

The Triple Warmer Channel of Hand-Shaoyang

Starting at the tip of the fourth finger, the Triple Warmer Channel crosses the back of the hand, and runs between the two bones of the forearm, and then up the back of the arm to the shoulder. It rises over the shoulder into the collarbone region, where it divides. One branch penetrates deeper, and meets the Triple Warmer. The other branch passes up through the nape and the ear, and ends at the outer edge of the eye. There are 23 acupoints along the Triple Warmer Channel.

Symptoms of disease in the Channel

Impairment of hearing, tinnitus, sore throat, eye pain and conjunctivitis, swelling of the cheeks, and local symptoms along the course of the Channel, such as pains in the shoulder, elbow, and arm.

The Ren Channel

This Channel originates in the lower abdomen. From the perineum it passes through the pubic region, and runs along the midline of the abdomen up to the throat. It then circles the mouth, and divides, each branch ending at the eyes. There are 24 acupoints this Channel.

Symptoms of disease in the Channel

Diseases of the Stomach and intestines, and problems of the reproductive organs, such as irregular menstruation, infertility, and emission.

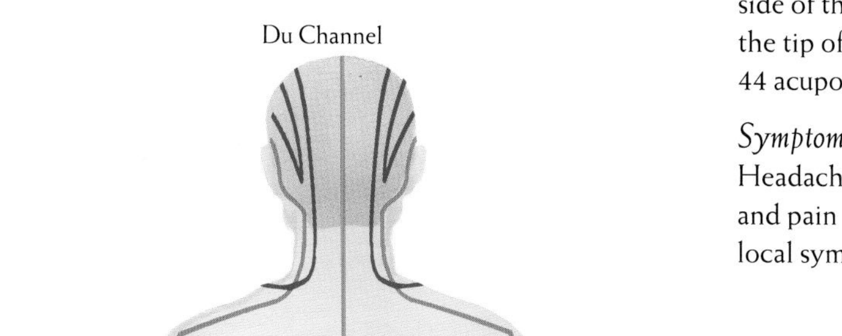

The Gall Bladder Channel of Foot-Shaoyang

This Channel starts at the outer eye socket and winds over the head. It then passes the nape, the 7th cervical vertebra, and the collarbone. The main Channel branches at the collarbone, and takes a zig-zag course down the side of the trunk. It then travels down the leg, and ends at the tip of the fourth toe. The Gall Bladder Channel has 44 acupoints along its course.

Symptoms of disease in the Channel

Headache, eye pain, bitterness in the mouth, swelling and pain in the collarbone and armpit regions, as well as local symptoms along the Channel's pathway.

The Liver Channel of Foot-Jueyin

Starting at the big toe, the Liver Channel passes over the top of the foot and ascends the inside of the leg to the groin. The Channel circles the genitals, and then follows a deeper path up through the abdomen, where it connects with the Liver and the Gall Bladder. It passes through the ribs, throat, nose, and eyes. It ends at the top of the head. There are 14 acupoints on the Liver Channel.

Symptoms of disease in the Channel

Tightness across the chest, hiccups, lumbago, hernia, menstrual problems, and urinary problems such as incontinence, and difficulty or pain in urination.

The Du Channel

This Channel starts in the lower abdomen. It emerges at the perineum, and travels upward through the spine. At the back of the neck, it enters the skull and connects with the brain. It then runs along the midline of the back of the head, to the forehead, nose, and upper lip. Its branches connect with the Kidney and the Heart. The Du Channel controls all the Yang Channels in the body. There are 28 acupoints along its course.

Symptoms of disease in the Channel

Spine and back pain, headache, impotence, emission, and infertility.

THE ACUPOINTS

THE FOLLOWING PAGES DESCRIBE THE LOCATION AND FUNCTION OF THE MOST COMMONLY USED ACUPOINTS. THE ACUPOINTS ARE USUALLY DESCRIBED ON ONE SIDE OF THE BODY, BUT REMEMBER MOST ARE PRESENT ON BOTH SIDES. REFER TO PAGES 32-3 FOR DETAILS ON USING THE ANATOMICAL "INCH" TO LOCATE ACUPOINTS, AND SEE PAGE 140 FOR THE BODY LANDMARKS DIAGRAMS.

Channel Abbreviations

The Channel names are abbreviated when used in the acupoint codes to indicate which Channel the point lies along (see also p. 10).

Lu	The Lung Channel
LI	The Large Intestine Channel
St	The Stomach Channel
Sp	The Spleen Channel
H	The Heart Channel
SI	The Small Intestine Channel
UB	The Urinary Bladder Channel
K	The Kidney Channel
P	The Pericardium Channel
T	The Triple Warmer Channel
GB	The Gall Bladder Channel
Liv	The Liver Channel
Du	The Du Channel
Ren	The Ren Channel
Extra	An extraordinary point

ACUPOINTS IN THE HEAD AND FACE REGION

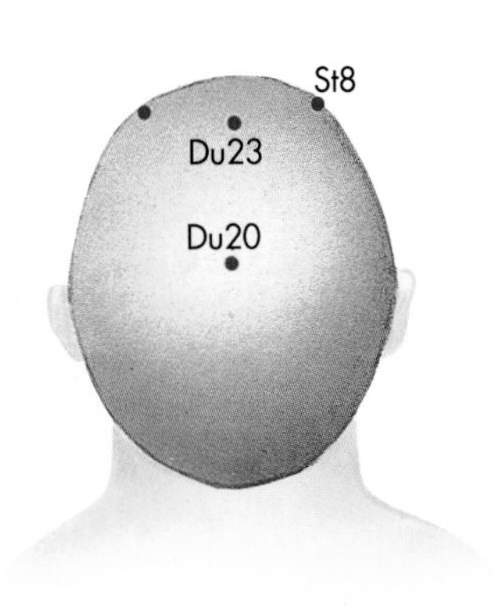

Du20 ~ Baihui
Location: on the top of the head, midway between the ears.
Application: headache, dizziness, tinnitus, amnesia, insomnia, and high blood pressure.

Du23 ~ Shangxing
Location: 1 inch behind the forehead hairline on the midline.
Application: headache, dizziness, tinnitus, amnesia, insomnia, and high blood pressure.

St8 ~ Touwei
Location: just inside the hairline at the corner of the forehead.
Application: headache, migraine, dizziness, and facial paralysis.

GB14 ~ Yangbai
Location: 1 inch above the eyebrow, directly in line with the pupil.
Application: headache, facial paralysis, and eye diseases.

Yintang (Extra)
Location: just above the nose, between the eyebrows.
Application: headache in the forehead, dizziness, high blood pressure, insomnia, eye diseases, rhinitis, and common cold.

UB2 ~ Zanzhu
Location: on the inner end of the eyebrow.
Application: headache, insomnia, eye diseases, and facial paralysis.

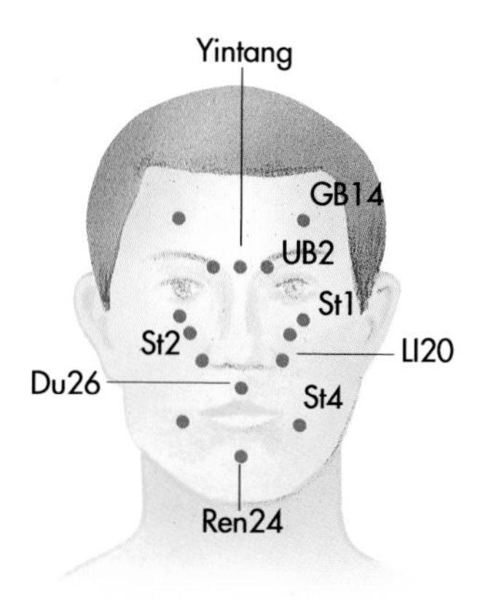

St1 ~ Chengqi
Location: directly below the pupil, on the lower edge of the eye socket.
Application: eye problems such as conjunctivitis, watery eyes, short-sight, long-sight, astigmatism, optic atrophy, optic neuritis, retinitis, and cataract.

St2 ~ Sibai
Location: the depression about 1 inch directly below the pupil.
Application: facial paralysis, trigeminal neuralgia, short-sight, and insomnia.

LI20 ~ Yingxiang
Location: at the base of the nose, either side of the nostrils.
Application: nasal obstruction, rhinitis, sinusitis, and facial paralysis.

Du26 ~ Renzhong
Location: in the furrow between the nose and the upper lip – ⅓ of the way toward the nose.
Application: stroke, shock, epilepsy, facial oedema, and acute lower back sprain.

St4 ~ Dicang
Location: just beyond the corner of the mouth, directly below the pupil.
Application: facial paralysis, trigeminal neuralgia, and toothache.

Ren24 ~ Chengjiang
Location: on the midline, below the lower lip in the crease of the chin.
Application: headache, toothache, and facial paralysis.

GB8 ~ Shuaigu
Location: 1.5 inches directly above the top of the ear.
Application: migraine (headache occurring on the side of the head).

Taiyang (Extra)
Location: on the temples, about 1 inch beyond the eye socket, on a line from the eye to the top of the ear.
Application: headache, migraine, dizziness, insomnia, eye diseases, facial paralysis, trigeminal neuralgia, high blood pressure, and common cold.

SI19 ~ Tinggong
Location: between the jaw joint and the front of the ear, in the depression formed when the mouth opens.
Application: tinnitus, age-related impaired hearing, dizziness, facial paralysis, and toothache.

GB2 ~ Tinghui
Location: between the jaw joint and the front of the ear, just below the depression formed when the mouth is open.
Application: tinnitus, age-related impaired hearing, dizziness, facial paralysis, and toothache.

St7 ~ Xiaguan
Location: the depression about 1 inch in front of the ear, found when the mouth shuts.
Application: toothache, facial paralysis, trigeminal neuralgia, spasm of the facial muscles, lower jaw pain, and tinnitus.

St6 ~ Jiache
Location: 1 inch diagonally up from the corner of the lower jaw.
Application: toothache, facial paralysis, trigeminal neuralgia, spasm of the facial muscles, lower jaw pain, and tinnitus.

T17 ~ Yifeng
Location: in the depression behind the ear lobe, between the mastoid process and the lower jaw.
Application: tinnitus, age-related impaired hearing, dizziness, eye diseases, headache, toothache, and facial paralysis.

Yiming (Extra)
Location: the depression below the mastoid process, 1 inch behind T17 (*Yifeng*).
Application: tinnitus, dizziness, headache, insomnia, long and short sight, night blindness, cataract, and optic atrophy.

Anmian (Extra)
Location: the midpoint between GB20 (*Fengchi*) and *Yiming* (Extra).
Application: insomnia, dizziness, and headache.

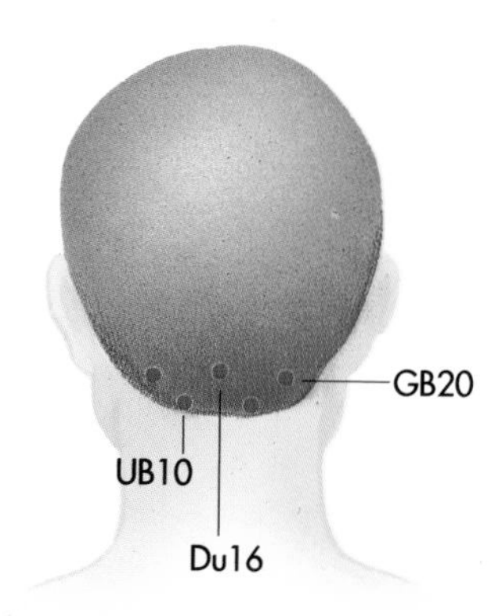

Du16 ~ Fengfu
Location: the hollow under the occipital protuberance on the midline, 1 inch above the hairline at the back of the head.
Application: headache, dizziness, high blood pressure, and neck pain.

GB20 ~ Fengchi
Location: at the base of the skull in the hollow in the hairline, between the mastoid process and the depression on the midline.
Application: common cold, headache, dizziness, eye diseases, high blood pressure, and insomnia.

UB10 ~ Tianzhu
Location: 0.5 inch above the hairline at the back of the head and 1.3 inches either side of the midline.
Application: occipital headache, stiffness and pain in the neck region.

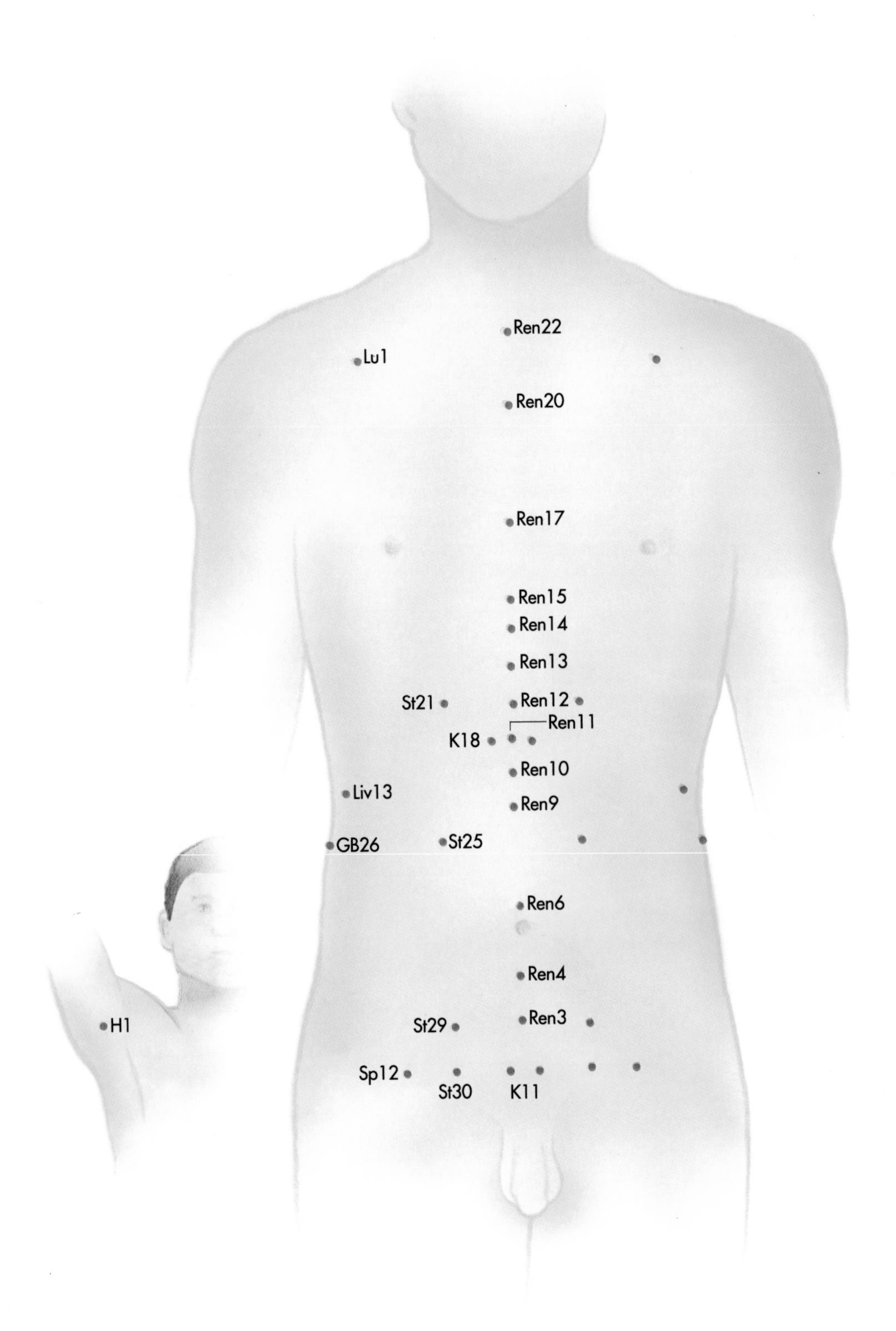

Ren22
Lu1
Ren20
Ren17
Ren15
Ren14
Ren13
St21
Ren12
Ren11
K18
Ren10
Liv13
Ren9
GB26
St25
Ren6
Ren4
H1
St29
Ren3
Sp12
St30
K11

ACUPOINTS IN THE ABDOMINAL REGION

Ren22 ~ Tiantu
Location: the hollow 0.5 inch above the top of the breastbone, on the midline.
Application: vomiting, asthma, bronchitis, and laryngitis.

Ren20 ~ Huagai
Location: 3 inches directly below the top of the breastbone, on the midline.
Application: asthma, coughs, and chest pain.

Lu1 ~ Zhongfu
Location: 1 inch below the collarbone at the shoulder end, and 6 inches either side of the midline.
Application: asthma, bronchitis, pneumonia, and pulmonary tuberculosis.

Ren17 ~ Tanzhong
Location: on the breastbone, midway between the nipples.
Application: coronary heart disease, chest pain, intercostal neuralgia, asthma, and vomiting.

Ren15 ~ Jiuwei
Location: 0.5 inch below the breastbone, on the midline of the belly.
Application: heart pain, stomachache, and vomiting.

Ren14 ~ Juque
Location: 6 inches above the navel, on the midline of the belly.
Application: palpitations, stomachache, and vomiting.

Ren13 ~ Shangwan
Location: 5 inches above the navel, on the midline of the belly.
Application: problems of the digestive system such as gastritis, peptic ulcers, vomiting, and abdominal distention.

Ren12 ~ Zhongwan
Location: 4 inches above the navel, on the midline of the belly.
Application: high blood pressure, neurosis, and problems of the digestive system such as stomachache, vomiting, indigestion, constipation, and abdominal distention.

St21 ~ Liangmen
Location: 4 inches above the navel and 2 inches either side of the midline of the belly.
Application: problems of the digestive system such as stomachache, indigestion, and bloating.

Ren11 ~ Jianli
Location: 3 inches above the navel, on the midline of the belly.
Application: stomachache, vomiting, indigestion, and general oedema.

K18 ~ Shiguan
Location: 3 inches above the navel and 0.5 inch either side of the midline.
Application: problems of the digestive system such as stomachache, abdominal pain, vomiting, and constipation.

Ren10 ~ Xiawan
Location: 2 inches above the navel, on the midline of the belly.
Application: stomachache, indigestion, and enteritis.

Liv13 ~ Zhangmen
Location: stand with your arms hanging down by your side and mark the point that your elbow reaches on each side.
Application: vomiting, bloating, diarrhoea, rib pain, and hepatic disease.

Ren9 ~ Shuifen
Location: 1 inch directly above the navel, on the midline of the belly.
Application: general oedema, diarrhoea, and abdominal pain.

St25 ~ Tianshu
Location: 2 inches either side of the navel.
Application: gastrointestinal diseases, abdominal pain, bloating, constipation, irregular menstruation, and painful periods.

GB26 ~ Daimai
Location: on the sides of the abdomen, directly below the armpit and level with the navel.
Application: enteritis, dysentery, intercostal neuralgia, cystitis, gynaecological diseases, irregular menstruation, and painful periods.

Ren6 ~ Qihai
Location: 1.5 inches below the navel, on the midline of the belly.
Application: abdominal pain, abdominal bloating, indigestion, emission, enuresis, irregular menstruation, painful periods, and neurosis.

Ren4 ~ Guanyuan
Location: 3 inches below the navel, on the midline of the belly.
Application: abdominal pain, diarrhoea, dysentery, irregular menstruation, painful periods, emission, enuresis, impotence, and urinary tract infections.

Ren3 ~ Zhongji
Location: 4 inches below the navel, on the midline of the belly.
Application: diseases of the urogenital system.

St29 ~ Guilai
Location: 4 inches below the navel and 2 inches either side of the midline of the belly.
Application: inflammation of the testicles (orchitis), inflammation of the female reproductive organs, and irregular menstruation.

K11 ~ Henggu
Location: 5 inches below the navel and 0.5 inch either side of the midline of the belly.
Application: hernia, emission, and impotence.

St30 ~ Qichong
Location: 5 inches below the navel and 2 inches either side of the midline of the belly.
Application: hernia, inflammation of the prostate gland (prostatitis), and irregular menstruation.

Sp12 ~ Chongmen
Location: 3.5 inches either side of the midline, on the same level as the upper margin of the pubic bone.
Application: abdominal pain and distension, back pain, and leg pain.

H1 ~ Jiquan
Location: the midpoint of the armpit.
Application: spine and shoulder pain, arm pain, paralysis of the arm, and numbness of the arm.

ACUPOINTS IN THE BACK REGION

GB21 ~ Jianjing
Location: on the top of the shoulder near the neck, midway between the 7th cervical vertebra and the outermost edge of the shoulder blade.
Application: neurosis, high blood pressure, stiff neck, shoulder pain, back pain, and hemiplegia.

Du14 ~ Dazhui
Location: on the back of the neck, between the 7th cervical and 1st thoracic vertebrae.
Application: common cold, fever, heatstroke, bronchitis, asthma, stiff neck, shoulder or back pain, paralysis, epilepsy, and psychosis.

SI15 ~ Jianzhongshu
Location: 2 inches either side of the midline of the back, level with the 7th cervical and 1st thoracic vertebrae.
Application: shoulder or back pain, stiff neck, bronchitis, and asthma.

UB12 ~ Fengmen
Location: 1.5 inches either side of the spine, level with the 2nd thoracic vertebra.
Application: common cold, fever, headache, cough, stiff neck, and back pain.

UB13 ~ Feishu
Location: 1.5 inches either side of the midline, level with the 3rd thoracic vertebra.
Application: bronchitis, pneumonia, tuberculosis of the lung, and common cold.

SI11 ~ Tianzong
Location: the midpoint of the shoulder blade.
Application: pain in the shoulder and scapular region, and numbness of the arm.

UB15 ~ Xinshu
Location: 1.5 inches either side of the spine, level with the 5th thoracic vertebra.
Application: palpitations, arrhythmia, angina pectoris, neurosis, hysteria, intercostal neuralgia, and back pain.

Du9 ~ Zhiyang
Location: between the 7th and 8th thoracic vertebrae, on the midline of the spine.
Application: hepatitis, inflammation of the gall bladder (cholecystitis), stomachache, angina pectoris, intercostal neuralgia, and back pain.

UB18 ~ Ganshu
Location: level with the 9th thoracic vertebra, 1.5 inches either side of the spine.
Application: eye diseases, hepatic disease, gastropathy, neurosis, intercostal neuralgia, and insomnia.

UB19 ~ Danshu
Location: level with the 10th thoracic vertebra, 1.5 inches either side of the spine.
Application: inflammation of the gall bladder (cholecystitis), hepatitis, back pain, sciatica, and intercostal neuralgia.

UB20 ~ Pishu
Location: level with the 11th thoracic vertebra, 1.5 inches either side of the spine.
Application: gastritis, enteritis, peptic ulcer, indigestion, hepatitis, general oedema, sciatica, and back pain.

UB21 ~ Weishu
Location: level with the 12th thoracic vertebra, 1.5 inches either side of the spine.
Application: gastritis, enteritis, peptic ulcer, indigestion, and hepatitis.

Du4 ~ Mingmen
Location: between the 2nd and 3rd lumbar vertebrae, on the midline of the spine.
Application: headache, tinnitus, lumbago, gynecological problems including irregular menstruation, and problems of the male reproductive system such as impotence, emission, and enuresis.

UB23 ~ Shenshu
Location: level with the 2nd lumbar vertebra, 1.5 inches either side of the spine.
Application: nephrosis, emission, enuresis, irregular menstruation, lumbago, tinnitus, insomnia, and general oedema.

Du3 ~ Yaoyangguan
Location: between the 4th and 5th lumbar vertebrae, on the midline of the spine.
Application: lower back pain, paralysis of the leg, irregular menstruation, emission, impotence, and enteritis.

UB25 ~ Dachangshu
Location: level with the 4th lumbar vertebra, 1.5 inches either side of the spine.
Application: enteritis, dysentery, constipation, sciatica, lumbago, lumbar muscle strain, paralysis and pain in sacroiliac joint.

Yaoyan (Extra)
Location: level with the 4th lumbar vertebra, about 4 inches either side of the spine.
Application: lumbago, sciatica, and problems with the female reproductive organs.

UB27 ~ Xiaochangshu
Location: level with the 1st sacral foramina, 1.5 inches either side of the spine.
Application: enuresis, emission, constipation, enteritis, pelvic inflammation, sciatica, lumbago, pain in sacroiliac joint.

UB31-34 ~ Baliao
Location: these 4 pairs of acupoints are located on the sacrum.
Application: lumbago, lower back pain, sciatica, paralysis, general oedema, irregular menstruation, and diseases of the urogenital system.

Du1 ~ Changqiang
Location: the midpoint between the coccyx and the anus.
Application: lower back pain, lumbago, enteritis, emission, proctoptosis, and haemorrhoids.

Jiaji (Extra)
Location: these 23 pairs of acupoints lie 0.5 inch either side of the spine, from the lower edge of the 1st cervical vertebra to the lower edge of the 5th lumbar vertebra.
Application: tuberculosis of the lung, asthma, diseases of the digestive system, diseases of the urogenital system, neurosis, paralysis, and back pain.

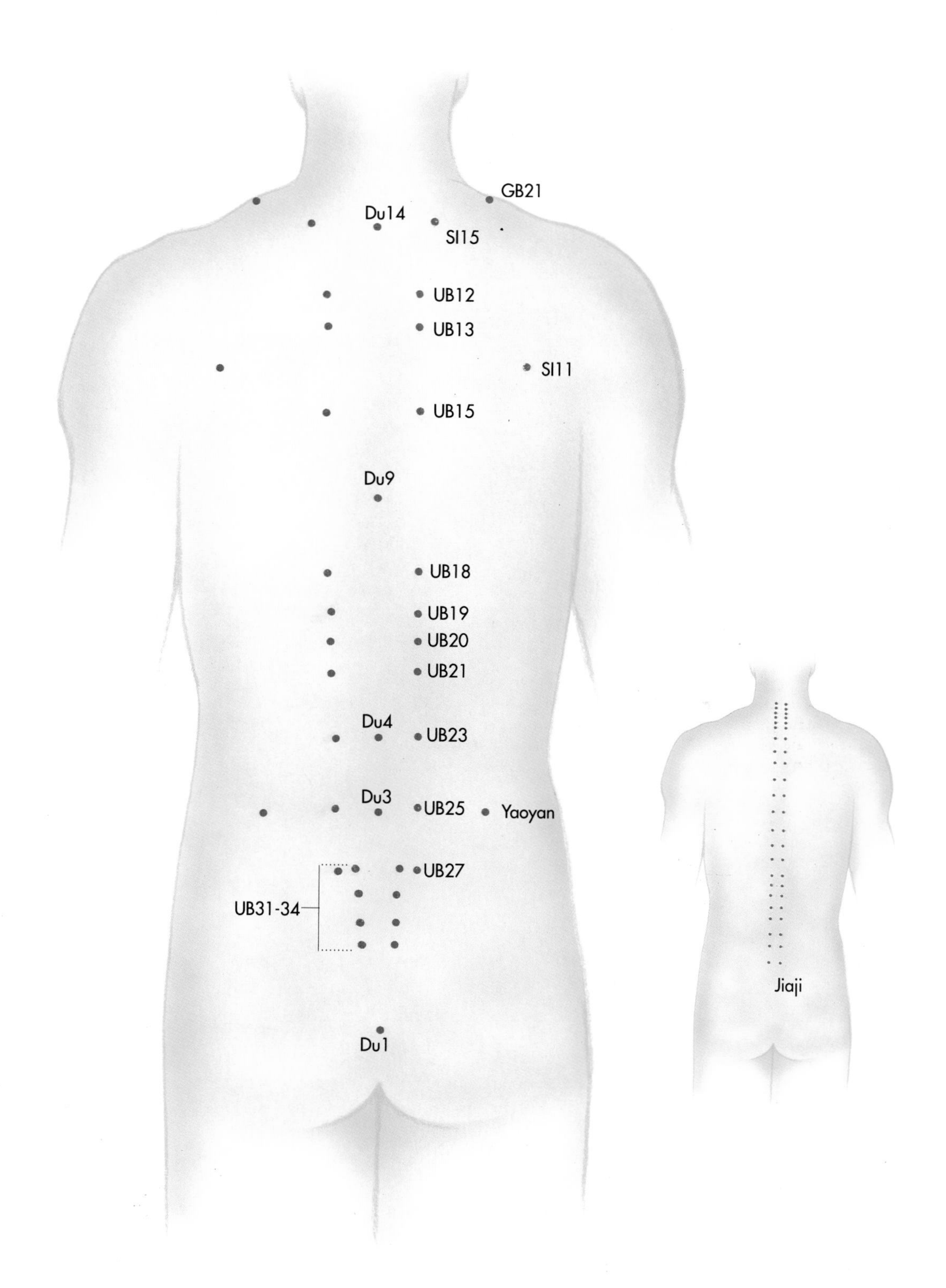
GB21
Du14
SI15
UB12
UB13
SI11
UB15
Du9
UB18
UB19
UB20
UB21
Du4
UB23
Du3
UB25
Yaoyan
UB27
UB31-34
Du1
Jiaji

ACUPOINTS IN THE ARM REGION

LI15 ~ Jianyu
Location: a dimple 2 inches below the outer edge of the shoulder, found when the arm is raised sideways.
Application: neck pain, shoulder pain, arm pain, and numbness in the arm.

Lu5 ~ Chize
Location: at the elbow crease, on the outside of the biceps tendon, found when the arm is slightly bent.
Application: asthma, cough, haemoptysis, sore throat, arm pain, and elbow-joint pain.

P3 ~ Quze
Location: at the elbow crease, on the inside of the biceps tendon, found when the arm is slightly bent.
Application: asthma, cough, haemoptysis, sore throat, arm pain, and elbow-joint pain.
Note: P3 is the key acupoint to treat sciatica.

H3 ~ Shaohai
Location: on the inside of the elbow crease.
Application: ulnar neuralgia and intercostal neuralgia.

P6 ~ Neiguan
Location: 2 inches from the wrist crease, in the middle of the inner forearm.
Application: heart diseases, chest pain, high blood pressure, abdominal pain, vomiting, headache, dizziness, hysteria, epilepsy, insomnia, shock, spine pain, and numbness of the arm.

Lu7 ~ Lieque
Location: 1.5 inches above the wrist crease, on the thumb-side of the inner forearm and just above the styloid process of the radius. Locate it by interlocking the thumbs and extending the index finger to reach it.
Application: headache, stiff neck, facial paralysis, cough, asthma, arm and wrist pain.

Lu9 ~ Taiyuan
Location: in the depression at the thumb-side of the wrist crease.
Application: cough, asthma, chest pain, arm and wrist pain.

P7 ~ Daling
Location: in the middle of the wrist crease on the inner forearm.
Application: heart disease, stomachache, chest pain, intercostal neuralgia, wrist pain, and insomnia.

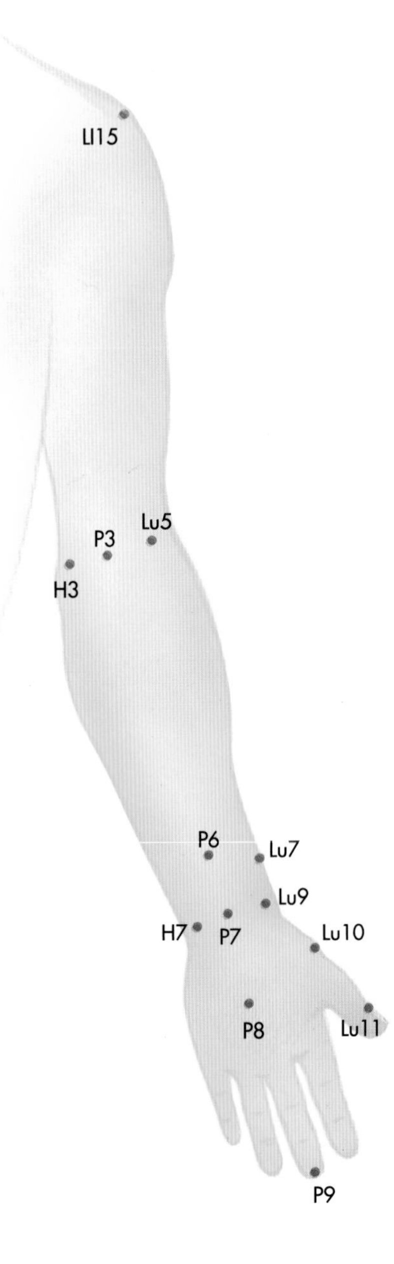

H7 ~ Shenmen
Location: on the ulnar end (little finger end) of the wrist crease.
Application: insomnia, dreaminess, hysteria, and palpitations.

Lu10 ~ Yuji
Location: 1.5 inches from the wrist crease, along the palm-side of the thumb, in the middle of the 1st metacarpal bone .
Application: cough, asthma, fever, and hand pain.

P8 ~ Laogong
Location: in the middle of the palm, between the 3rd and 4th metacarpal bones.
Application: chest and rib pain, headache, dizziness, heat stroke, and hysteria.

Lu11 ~ Shaoshang
Location: 0.1 inch from the outside corner (radial surface) of the thumbnail bed.
Application: cough and sore throat.

P9 ~ Zhongchong
Location: at the tip of the middle finger.
Application: headache, tinnitus, and angina pectoris.

T14 ~ Jianliao
Location: the dimple below the edge of the shoulder on the back of the body, about 1 inch behind LI15 (*Jianyu*).
Application: spine pain, neck and shoulder pain, arm pain, and paralysis of the arm.

SI9 ~ Jianzhen
Location: 1 inch above the end of the posterior armpit crease.
Application: shoulder pain, paralysis of the arm, tinnitus, and impaired hearing.

LI14 ~ Binao
Location: at the lower end of the deltoid muscle on the back of the arm, found when the arm is raised.
Application: neck pain, shoulder pain, arm pain, paralysis and numbness of the arm.

LI12 ~ Zhouliao
Location: 1 inch diagonally above the radial end (thumb side) of the elbow crease on the back of the arm, found when the arm is bent.
Application: stiff neck, arm pain, elbow pain, and arthritis.

LI11 ~ Quchi
Location: at the radial end (thumb side) of the elbow crease, found when the arm is bent.
Application: arm pain, paralysis of the arm, muscular atrophy of the arm, high blood pressure, headache, dizziness, and neck pain.

SI8 ~ Xiaohai
Location: the depression in the back of the elbow, found when the arm is bent.
Application: stiff neck, shoulder pain, and back pain.

LI10 ~ Shousanli
Location: 2 inches down from the radial end (thumb side) of the elbow crease.
Application: arm pain, paralysis of the arm, abdominal pain, diarrhoea, headache, and toothache.

T6 ~ Zhigou
Location: 3 inches above the midpoint of the wrist on the back of the forearm.
Application: shoulder pain, arm pain, and constipation.

T5 ~ Waiguan
Location: 2 inches above the midpoint of the wrist, on the back of the forearm.
Application: arm pain, paralysis of the arm, tinnitus, impaired hearing, stiff neck, and hemiplegia.

T4 ~ Yangchi
Location: the dimple in the middle of the wrist on the back of the hand.
Application: wrist pain, arm pain, headache, common cold, and fever.

LI5 ~ Yangxi
Location: the hollow on the wrist, just off the base of the thumb, found when the thumb points upward.
Application: wrist pain, headache, tinnitus, and toothache.

LI4 ~ Hegu
Location: on the back of the hand in the web between the thumb and index finger.
Application: headache, toothache, sore throat, impaired hearing, eye diseases, rhinitis, facial paralysis, arm pain, paralysis of the arm, neurosis, common cold, and fever.
Note: LI4 is the key acupoint for treating headaches and toothache.

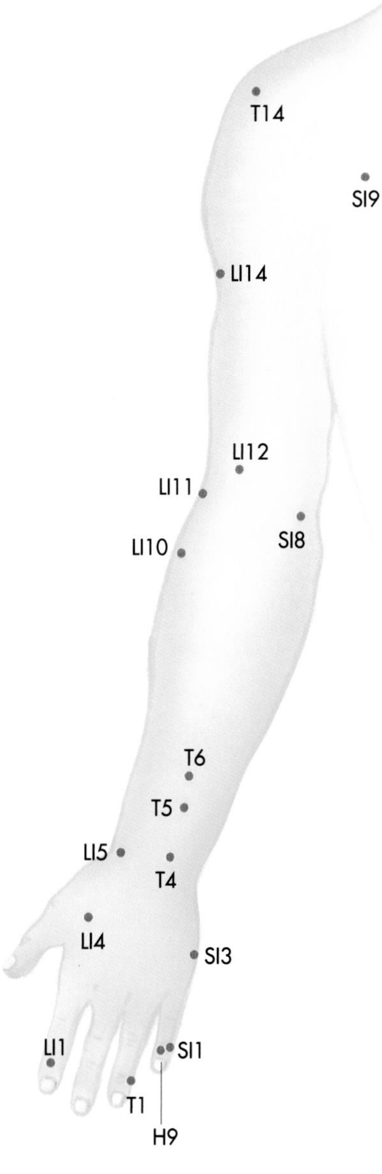

SI3 ~ Houxi
Location: at the end of the palm crease, on the ulnar side of the hand, found when the fist is slightly clenched.
Application: headache in either the top or back of the head, stiff neck, shoulder pain, back pain, and intercostal neuralgia.

LI1 ~ Shangyang
Location: 0.1 inch from the corner of the index fingernail, on the radial side (thumb side).
Application: toothache, sore throat, shoulder pain, and numbness of the arm.

T1 ~ Guanchong
Location: 0.1 inch from the corner of the fourth fingernail, on the ulnar side.
Application: headache, sore throat, and arm pain.

H9 ~ Shaochong
Location: 0.1 inch from the corner of the little fingernail, on the radial side (thumb side).
Application: palpitations, chest pain, and stroke.

SI1 ~ Shaoze
Location: 0.1 inch from the corner of the little fingernail, on the ulnar side.
Application: headache and eye diseases.

Baxie (Extra)
Location: 4 acupoints are located between the knuckles on the back of the hand, found when the fist is loosely clenched.
Application: hand pain, finger-joint pain, headache, toothache, sore throat, and neck pain.

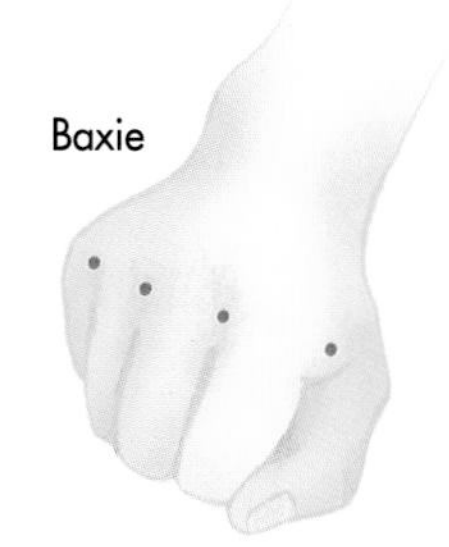

ACUPOINTS IN THE LEG REGION

St31 ~ Biguan

Location: on the line between the kneecap and the pelvic bone, level with the genital region.
Application: hip and leg pain, paralysis and numbness of the leg, and prolapsed lumbar intervertebral disc.

St32 ~ Futu

Location: 6 inches above the top of the kneecap, in line with its outside edge.
Application: paralysis of the leg, and neuritis of the lateral cutaneous nerve of the thigh.

St34 ~ Liangqiu

Location: 2 inches above the top of the kneecap, in line with its outside edge.
Application: stomachache, diarrhoea, mastitis, and knee pain.

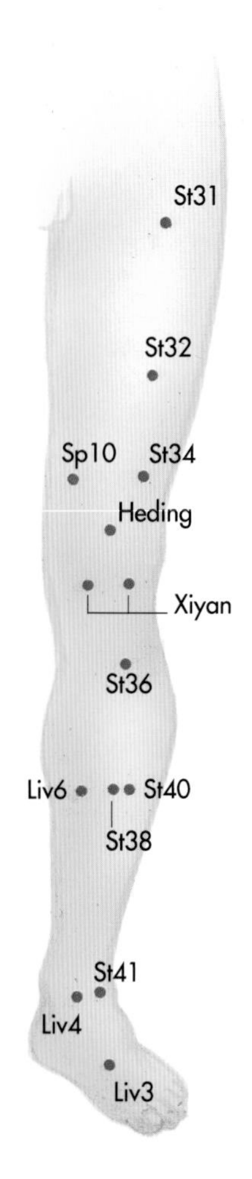

Sp10 ~ Xuehai

Location: 2 inches above the top of the kneecap, in line with its inside edge.
Application: irregular menstruation, dysfunctional uterine bleeding, and urticaria.

Heding (Extra)

Location: the depression on the upper edge of the kneecap, found when the leg is bent.
Application: knee pain and leg pain.

Xiyan (Extra)

Location: these 2 acupoints are located in the 2 depressions of the knee joint, just below the kneecap, found when the leg is bent. The acupoint on the medial side is called inner *Xiyan* and the one on the lateral side is outer *Xiyan* or St35.
Application: knee and lower leg pain.

St36 ~ Zusanli

Location: 3 inches below the kneecap, on the outside of the leg.
Application: diseases of the digestive system, neurosis, high blood pressure, lumbago, leg pain, paralysis or numbness of the leg, and hemiplegia.
Note: St36 is very effective for relieving abdominal pain.

St40 ~ Fenglong

Location: 8 inches above the outside ankle joint.
Application: headache, dizziness, sore throat, stomachache, diarrhoea, oedema of the leg, and hemiplegia.

St38 ~ Tiaokou

Location: on the outside of the leg, midway between the kneecap and the ankle joint.
Application: arthritis of the knee, paralysis of the leg, and shoulder pain.
Note: St38 is the key acupoint for relieving shoulder pain.

Liv6 ~ Zhongdu

Location: 7 inches above the inside ankle joint.
Application: pain in the leg joints.

St41 ~ Jiexi

Location: the depression in the middle of the front of the ankle joint, between the tendons.
Application: headache, sprained ankle, and foot drop.

Liv4 ~ Zhongfeng

Location: the depression 1 inch in front of the inside ankle joint and by the tendon.
Application: lower abdominal pain, penis pain, and emission.

Liv3 ~ Taichong

Location: on the top of the foot, in the furrow between the 1st and 2nd toes, where the bones merge.
Application: headache, dizziness, high blood pressure, insomnia, irregular menstruation, painful periods, sciatica, paralysis, and foot pain.

UB36 ~ Chengfu

Location: the midpoint of the crease below the buttock.
Application: lumbago, sciatica, leg pain, numbness of the leg, paralysis, constipation, and haemorrhoids.

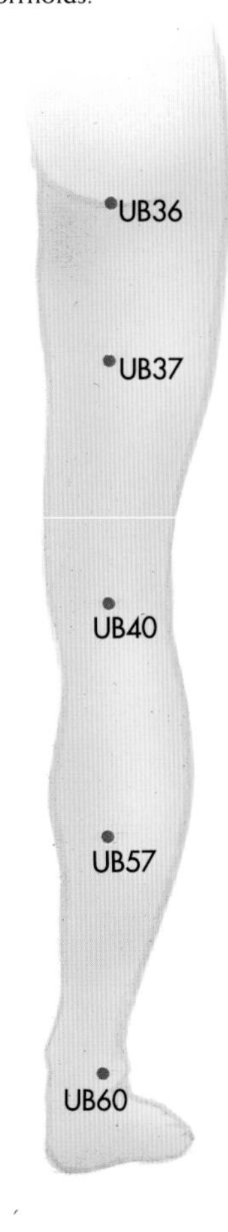

UB37 ~ Yinmen
Location: 6 inches below the crease of the buttock, in the middle of the back of the leg.
Application: lumbago, sciatica, leg pain, numbness and paralysis of the leg, constipation, and haemorrhoids.

UB40 ~ Weizhong
Location: the midpoint of the knee crease at the back of the leg.
Application: lumbago, prolapse of lumbar intervertebral disc, sciatica, numbness and paralysis of the leg, hemiplegia, and arthritis of the knee.
Note: UB40 is very effective in relieving lower back pain.

UB57 ~ Chengshan
Location: in the middle of the back of the calf, midway between the knee crease and the heel.
Application: lumbago, prolapse of lumbar intervertebral disc, sciatica, paralysis, numbness of the leg, spasm of the lower leg muscles, and haemorrhoids.

UB60 ~ Kunlun
Location: on the outside of the ankle joint, midway between the ankle bone and the Achilles tendon.
Application: headache, stiff neck and back, back pain, lumbago, sciatica, paralysis, ankle sprain, and heel pain.

GB30 ~ Huantiao
Location: on the side of the buttocks, two thirds of the way toward the top of the thigh bone from the sacrum.
Application: lumbago, hip and leg pain, and paralysis of the leg.

GB31 ~ Fengshi
Location: the point on the outside of the thigh that the tip of your middle finger reaches if you stand with your arms hanging down by your sides.
Application: leg pain, paralysis of the leg, and sciatica.

GB34 ~ Yanglingquan
Location: on the outside of the lower leg in a depression just in front of and a little below the head of the fibula.
Application: hepatic diseases, gall bladder problems, high blood pressure, intercostal neuralgia, shoulder pain, lumbago, numbness or paralysis of the leg, and knee pain.

Dannangdian (Extra)
Location: about 1 inch below GB34 (*Yanglingquan*).
Application: gall bladder problems.

GB39 ~ Xuanzhong
Location: 3 inches above the outside ankle bone in the front of the fibula.
Application: knee or ankle pain, chest pain, stiff neck, and hemiparalysis.

GB40 ~ Qiuxu
Location: the depression diagonally below the outside ankle bone.
Application: chest pain, ankle pain, sciatica, and gall bladder inflammation.

Liv8 ~ Ququan
Location: on the inner end of the crease at the back of the knee.
Application: abdominal pain, diarrhoea, diseases of the reproductive organs, back and leg pain, and knee pain.

Sp9 ~ Yinlingquang
Location: below the knee joint in the depression between the tibia and the calf muscle, on the inside lower leg.
Application: diseases of the urogenital system, abdominal pain, general oedema, lumbago, and paralysis or numbness of the leg.

Sp6 ~ Sanyinjiao
Location: 3 inches above the inside ankle joint, just behind the tibia.
Application: diseases of the reproductive system, abdominal pain, diarrhoea, general oedema, sciatica, lumbago, leg pain, and paralysis of the leg.

K3 ~ Taixi
Location: midway between the inside ankle joint and the Achilles tendon.
Application: diseases of the urogenital system, insomnia, lumbago, sciatica, leg pain, and paralysis of the leg.

K6 ~ Zhaohai
Location: the depression 1 inch below the top of the inside ankle joint.
Application: menstrual disorders and neurosis.

Sp4 ~ Gongsun
Location: on the inside arch of the foot, about 1 inch behind the long bone of the big toe.
Application: stomachache, indigestion, vomiting, diarrhoea, and painful periods.

K1 ~ Yongquan
Location: on the midline of the sole of the foot, between the 2nd and 3rd metatarsal bones.
Application: headache, high blood pressure, insomnia, heat stroke, shock, cerebral haemorrhage, sciatica, lumbago, paralysis of the leg, leg and foot pain.

GB30
GB31
Liv8
Sp9
GB34
Dannangdian
Sp6
K3
K6
GB39
Sp4
GB40

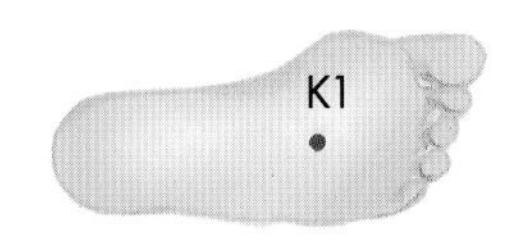

THE PAIN-RELIEF POINTS

THE MAIN FUNCTIONS OF PAIN-RELIEF POINTS ARE TO RELIEVE PAIN AND TREAT DISORDERS OF CERTAIN ORGANS AND REGIONS (SEE P. 12). APPLY DEEP AND FIRM PRESSURE TO THESE POINTS DURING TREATMENT.

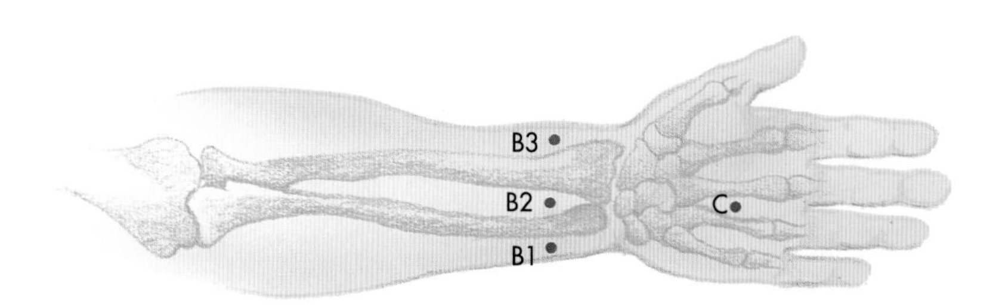

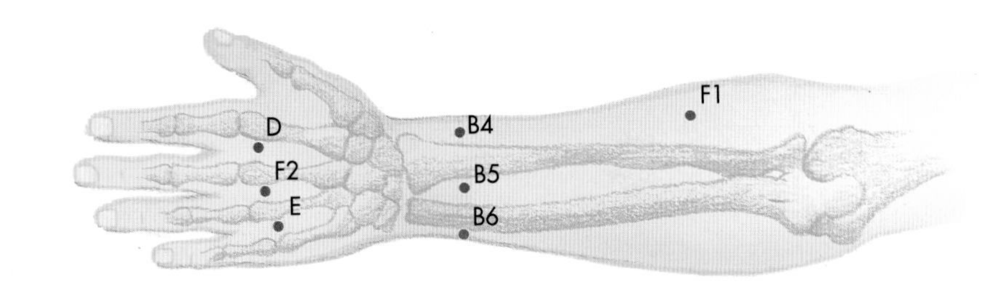

Point B1

Location: 2 inches above the wrist crease on the ulnar side of the inner forearm.
Application: frontal headache, eye pain, frontal toothache, sore throat, stomach-ache.

Point B2

Location: 2 inches above the wrist crease, in the middle of the lower forearm. This is the same position as P3 (*Neiguan*).
Application: toothache and chest pain.

Point B3

Location: 2 inches above the wrist crease on the radial side of the inner forearm.
Application: chest pain and high blood pressure.

Point B4

Location: 2 inches above the wrist crease on the back of the arm on the radial side.
Application: headache (in the top of the head), jaw pain, shoulder pain, and sore sides.

Point B5

Location: 2 inches above the midpoint of the wrist, on the back of the forearm. This is the same position as T5 (*Waiguan*).
Application: neck, shoulder, upper back, arm, elbow, wrist, and finger pain.

Point B6

Location: 2 inches above the wrist on the back of the forearm, on the ulnar side.
Application: occipital headache (in the back of the head), pain in the cervical and thoracic vertebrae.

Point C

Location: between the 3rd and 4th metacarpal bones in the palm, and just by P8 (*Laogong*).
Application: toothache.

Point D

Location: behind the 2nd and 3rd metacarpophalangeal joints on the back of the hand.
Application: cervical spondylopathy and stiff neck.

Point E

Location: behind the 4th and 5th metacarpophalangeal joints on the back of the hand.
Application: sciatica and hip pain.

Point F1

Location: between LI11 (*Quchi*) and T4 (*Yangchi*), ¼ of the way toward LI11.
Application: lower back pain and lumbar sprain.

Point F2

Location: behind the 3rd and 4th metacarpophalangeal joints on the back of the hand.
Application: lower back pain and lumbar sprain.

There are 12 A pain-relief points lying on the radial border of the 2nd metacarpal bone. Each one has a specific application.

Point A1
Relieves painful disorders of the head, eyes, ears, nose, and mouth.

Point A2
Relieves neck pain and sore throat.

Point A3
Relieves pain from the shoulder, elbow, wrist, hand, and arm.

Point A4
Helps to treat disorders of the Heart, Lungs, chest, upper back, and bronchus.

Point A5
Benefits the Liver and Gall Bladder.

Point A6
Helps to treat disorders of the Stomach and Spleen.

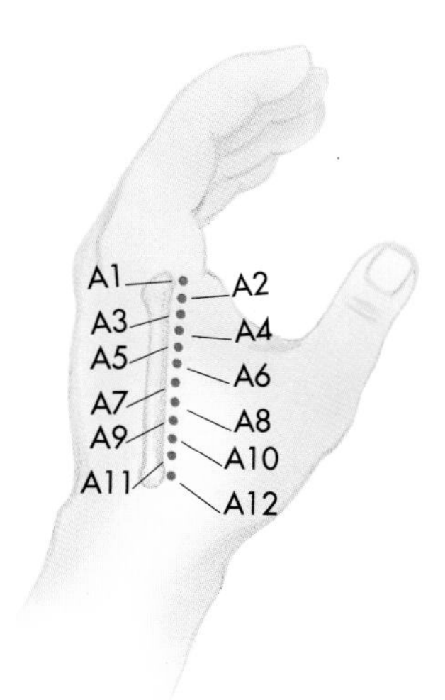

Point A7
Helps to treat disorders of the duodenum and the Small Intestine.

Point A8
Helps to treat disorders of the Kidneys, Large Intestine, and Small Intestine.

Point A9
Helps to treat disorders of the lower back, abdomen, Large and Small Intestine.

Point A10
Helps to treat disorders of the lower abdomen, uterus, Urinary Bladder, rectum, anus, appendix, and the urogenital system.

Point A11
Benefits the leg and knee.

Point A12
Helps to treat foot and ankle pain.

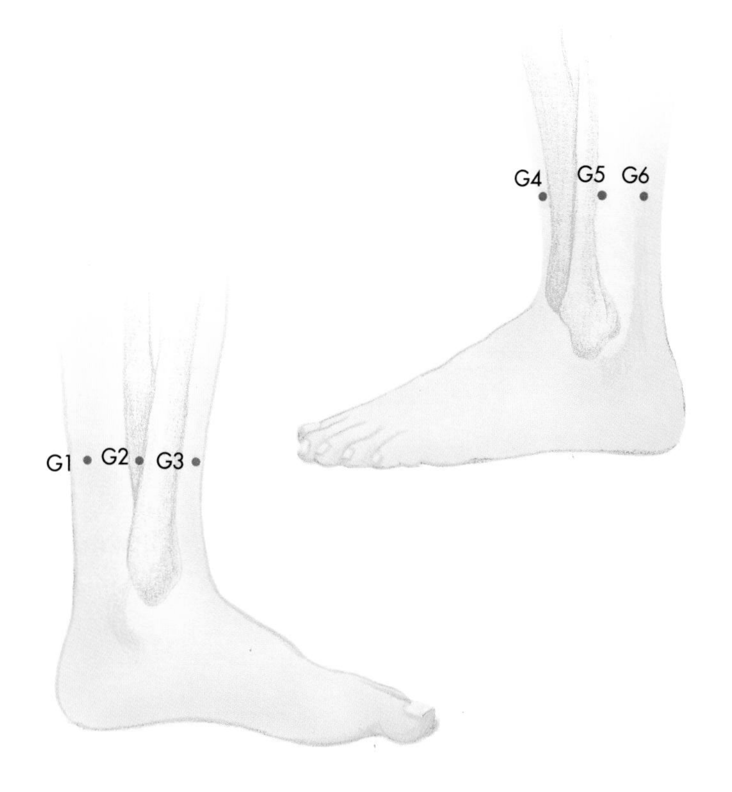

Point G1
Location: 2.5 inches above the inside ankle joint at the anterior border of the tendon.
Application: abdominal pain, abdominal distension, painful periods, and heel pain.

Point G2
Location: 2.5 inches above the inside ankle.
Application: sore sides.

Point G3
Location: 2.5 inches above the inside ankle joint at the anterior border of the tibia.
Application: knee pain.

Point G4
Location: 2.5 inches above the outside ankle at the anterior border of the fibula.
Application: leg muscle pain, knee and foot pain.

Point G5
Location: 2.5 inches above the lateral ankle joint at the posterior border of the fibula.
Application: pain in the lower side, hip pain, and ankle pain.

Point G6
Location: 2.5 inches above the outside ankle at the anterior border of the tendon.
Application: lower back pain, sciatica, leg muscle spasm, and foot pain.

BODY LANDMARKS

USE THE ILLUSTRATIONS BELOW TO HELP YOU IDENTIFY THE MAIN BONES AND ANATOMICAL FEATURES THAT ARE USED AS BODY LANDMARKS FOR LOCATING ACUPOINTS (SEE ALSO PP. 32-3).

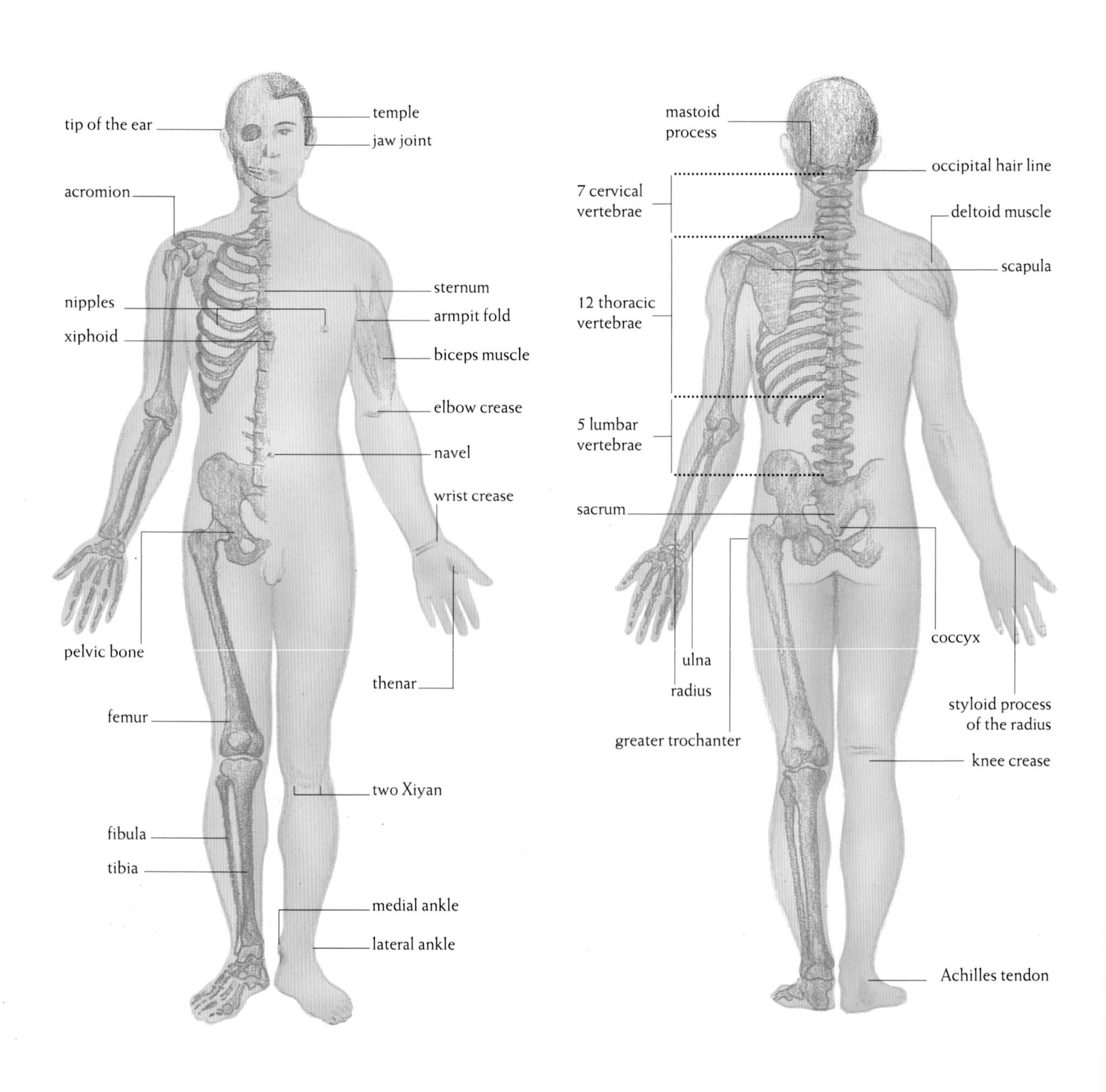

GLOSSARY

The language of Chinese medicine is beyond simple translation. Some terms such as Qi, Yin and Yang are becoming accepted in the West, and in time you will become familiar with more terms. Use this glossary to look up the key terms used in the book, and refer to the Introduction (see pp. 8-13) for a fuller explanation of the theory of Chinese medicine.

acupoint
Hundreds of acupoints, known as normal acupoints, lie along the course of the Channels and help to transmit Qi and blood through the Channels. They are referred to by code names and a Chinese name (see p. 13). Other acupoints, known as extraordinary acupoints, do not lie on any of the Channels.

acute
Describes a disease or condition that has a rapid onset and severe symptoms.

anterior
The front of the body when standing in the upright position.

blood
This Chinese term is identifiable as the substance the West calls blood, but it is not exactly the same. It flows not only through the blood vessels, but also through the Channels. Blood helps to generate Qi, and usually flows with Qi in the Channels (see pp. 8-9).

Channels
The Channels are the unseen pathways that carry Qi and blood through the body (see pp. 10-11). They link with each other to form a network that connects the Viscera, and all parts of the body. They also link the interior of the body to the exterior – the Viscera to the surface. There are 12 Regular Channels, 8 extra Channels, and some collaterals. The Channels are sometimes called Meridians.

Channel blockage
see Qi-blood stagnation

Channel disturbance
This occurs when Qi-blood flow has been upset. It is caused by an invasion of external or internal factors. The external pathogenic factors are the Six Evils. The internal factors include an irregular lifestyle, exhaustion, or an excess of one of the Seven Extreme Emotions – over-excitement, anger, anxiety, worry, grief, fear, and shock. Channel disturbance results in Qi-blood stagnation.

chronic
Describes a persistent or recurring condition, often of long duration. Conditions may start as acute and become chronic if untreated.

Extraordinary acupoint (extra)
An acupoint that is not located on a Channel. These points do not have a code name; just their Chinese name is used, for example *Taiyang*.

Extra Channel
Unlike the Regular Channels, these 8 Channels are not associated with organs. Du and Ren are the commonly used ones.

inch
An anatomical measurement used in Chinese medicine to help locate acupoints on the body (see pp. 32-3). Not to be confused with the imperial inch.

lateral
The outer side, for example the lateral ankle is the outside of the ankle.

major acupoints
These are simply acupoints that are given emphasis in the opening the Channels sequences. They are selected according to the condition being treated. The major acupoints should be pressed a few more times than other acupoints in a sequence.

medial
The inner side, for example the medial ankle is the inside of the ankle.

midline
An imaginary line which runs through the centre of the body.

pain-pressure point
The central point of an area of pain. The pain-pressure point is regarded as a type of pain-relief point.

pain-relief point
These have the specific function of relieving pain in certain parts of the body. Generally, deep, firm pressure is required for their manipulation.

posterior
The back of the body when in the upright position.

Qi
Pronounced "chee" (as in cheetah), an essential substance needed to support life. In a narrow sense, it is vital energy. Qi nourishes the body and protects it from external damage (see pp. 8-9).

Qi-blood flow
The circulation of Qi and blood in the Channels. Qi and blood support and complement each other: blood needs Qi to keep it moving, and Qi needs blood to generate it (see pp. 8-9). In health, Qi and blood flow smoothly through the Channels.

Qi-blood stagnation
Qi and blood stagnate in the Channels and block them, as a result of Channel disturbance. This is referred to as Channel blockage, or Qi-blood stagnation. Symptoms of Channel disturbance, such as pain, may be apparent in certain parts of the body.

Regular Channels
There are 12 Regular Channels. Each one is associated with a particular organ, runs along either the arm or the leg, and is either Yin or Yang (see pp. 10-11). Each Regular Channel has bilateral symmetry.

Six Evils
These are Cold, Damp, Dryness, Fire, Summer-heat, and Wind. They are the external pathogenic factors that can upset Qi-blood flow in the Channels. This happens when any one or more of the Six Evils is either in excess, or in insufficient supply (see p. 9).

Symptoms
Symptoms and signs of disease, such as pain, can be seen as part of a pattern, manifesting Qi-blood disturbance in particular Channels. They can reflect either a problem in the corresponding organ or a disturbance along the course of one of the Channels.

Viscera
This term refers to three groups of organs (see p. 9): the Zang organs, which are Yin; the Fu organs, which are Yang; and the Extraordinary organs.

Yin and Yang
Yin and Yang create life by touching each other: they are the basis of all life. They are the opposite aspects of matter and phenomena in nature, but they are complementary and interdependent. For complete health and wellbeing, the two forces need to be in perfect balance in the body (see p. 8).

INDEX

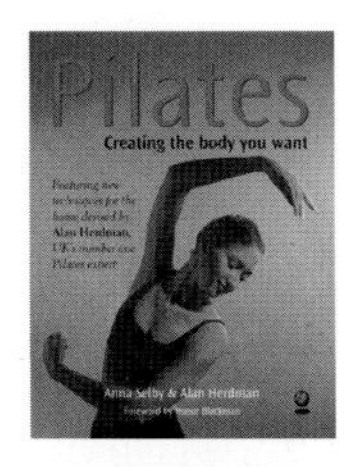

Pilates

Anna Selby & Alan Herdman ISBN 1 85675 115 5 £12.99
Mind-body exercise routines to tone muscles, lengthen limbs and improve posture.

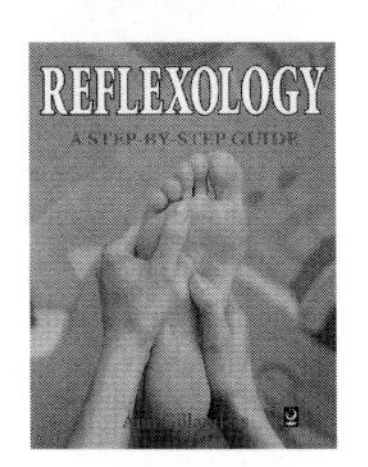

Reflexology: A step-by-step guide

Ann Gillanders ISBN 185675 081 7 £11.99
Treatments for the hands and feet to relieve pain and combat ailments.

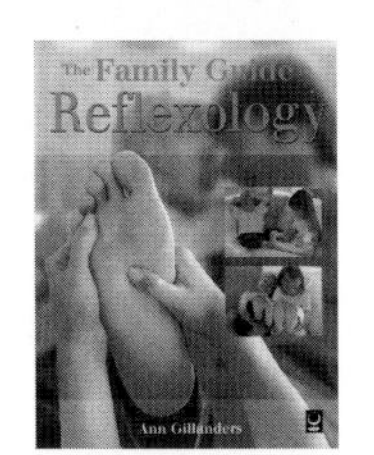

The Family Guide to Reflexology

Ann Gillanders ISBN 1 85675 049 3 £11.99
Offers treatments for all the family, covering a wide range of ailments.

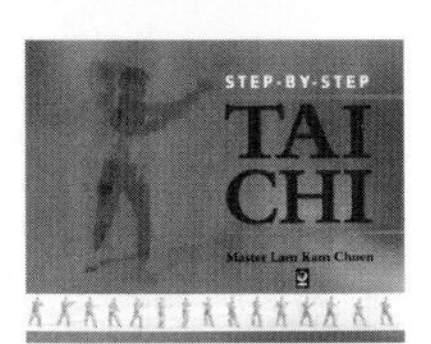

Step-by-Step Tai Chi

Master Lam Kam Chuen ISBN 1 85675 066 3 £11.99
Meditation combined with exercises, to soothe the mind and uplift the spirit.

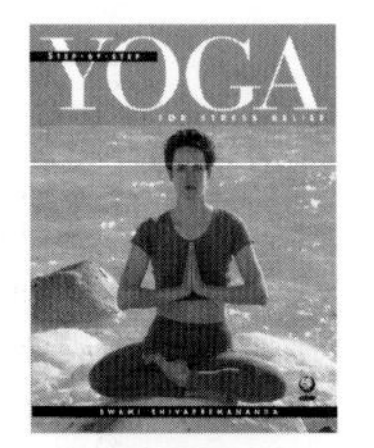

Yoga for Stress Relief

Swami Shivapremananda ISBN 1 85675 126 0 £11.99
Yoga positions, exercises and meditations to relieve and prevent stress.

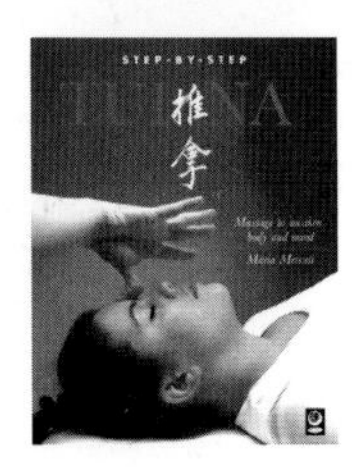

Step-by-Step Tui Na

Maria Mercati ISBN 1 85675 044 2 £11.99
Energising massage and manipulation from Traditional Chinese Medicine.

To order titles featured on this page or to request a catalogue of titles published by Gaia Books please call 01453 752985, fax 01453 752987 or write to Gaia Books Ltd, 20 High Street, Stroud, Glos GL5 1AZ
e-mail:sales@gaiabooks.co.uk web site: www.gaiabooks.co.uk